PHILOSOPHICAL H

PHILOSOPHICAL PROBLEMS

LEONARD GODDARD

Professor of Logic and Metaphysics
University of St. Andrews

SCOTTISH ACADEMIC PRESS

EDINBURGH

Published by
Scottish Academic Press Ltd,
33 Montgomery Street
Edinburgh EH7 5JX

SBN 7073 0136 X

© 1977 Scottish Academic Press Ltd

Printed in Great Britain by
R. & R. Clark Ltd, Edinburgh

CONTENTS

for
Phyl, Sue and Jane

PREFACE

This is a book for newcomers to philosophy, though I have made no
attempt to say what philosophy is or what makes a problem philosophical. I believe the only way to find out what philosophy is, is to
do it rather than talk about it. But perhaps I should say here that
what motivates a good deal of philosophical enquiry is that there
often seems to be a gap between many of the ordinary beliefs we
have and the evidence we have for them. And since the beliefs are
not ones which we usually want to give up, a lot of philosophical
discussion turns on the question of whether or not the gap can be
filled. Sometimes the answer seems to be no, and there is then a
tendency to become sceptical about the belief; sometimes it seems to
be yes. But whether yes or no, the answer is scarcely ever conclusive.
Whatever argument is put up, there is almost always a counter
argument; and sometimes an argument is put forward in the hope
that someone else may be able to find a reply to it. The moral in this
for beginners is that philosophy should not be read as fact or as
established theory; and no argument should be allowed to go un-
challenged. However convincing a particular argument may appear
to be, the chances are that there is some nasty hole in it somewhere.
To philosophise is to find the holes and to plug them or dig them
deeper.

Whatever philosophy is, it is not a subject with a beginning,
middle and end. So I have not attempted to write a continuous
narrative. I have simply chosen six problems, which have fascinated
many generations of philosophers, and considered them independently. There is, however, a linking theme, the problem of cause and
effect. This is the topic of the first chapter. The remaining chapters
depend on the first to some extent, but not very much on each other,
and I hope it will be possible for readers to jump straight to topics
which interest them most. There may, however, be some advantage
in taking things as they come.

It would have been nice in a book intended for beginners to have
presented half-a-dozen easy problems as a gentle introduction. But
easy problems would have been solved long ago and would have
lost their fascination. The only way of learning how to swim in

philosophical waters is to be thrown in at the deep end. There are, too, limitations on the extent to which the problems can be made easily understandable, as distinct from being made easy. I have tried to overcome these limitations by leaving out both recent technical developments and historical background. This last may seem surprising since the origins of every philosophical problem can be found in the history of the subject and one might expect that when a problem first arises it does so in a simple form. This is not always so, however; and in any case, to raise a problem in its historical context almost always raises extraneous subsidiary questions of a scholarly or textual nature. But of course I have drawn freely on historical examples and arguments and my debts will be obvious to anyone familiar with the subject or to anyone who follows up the suggested reading at the end. For the beginner, however, it is not necessary to know anything about the history of the subject in order to do philosophy, though it is necessary in order to do it well. What I hope is that those who start their philosophy with this book will be stimulated to turn to the history to find out more. They will then discover philosophising at its best.

I am grateful to the Australian National University for appointing me to a Fellowship which gave me the opportunity to write this book, among other things, and to the University of St. Andrews for giving me leave to take it up. On a more personal level, I wish to express my gratitude to Professors D. M. Armstrong, S. C. Haydon and J. A. Passmore, each of whom read an early draft and gave me much valuable advice.

L.G.

St. Andrews
and Canberra

Chapter 1

CAUSE AND EFFECT

Things happen; and we ask why. Or things which we expect to happen, do not; and again we ask why. It seems natural for us always to seek a reason or explanation for any change which takes place or for the non-occurrence of any expected change which fails to take place. And in many cases, it is not only natural that we seek an explanation but important that we find one. If an aeroplane crashes, we might find, after a long investigation, that it was the fault of the pilot; or we might find that it was due to an engine failure. In such cases the answer to the question 'Why?' is important to a great many people because it is on the basis of the answer that we apportion responsibility, blame, damages and punishment.

At a different level of importance, if we know why certain things happen, we may be able to bring about desired ends and prevent undesirable ones. We may be able to control events. It is because Jenner noticed that people who handle cows do not usually get small-pox, and came up with the right answer to the question why, that he was able to interfere in the course of nature and prevent the occurrence of smallpox by infecting potential sufferers with cowpox. In almost every aspect of our lives we exercise control over our environment. We anticipate and interfere in order to make things happen or to prevent other things from happening. We take pills; we wear spectacles to correct our vision and clothes to keep us warm; we use insecticides, pulleys, levers, tools and engines; we put sails on yachts and petrol in the car; we water plants and feed animals; we sow in the spring in the expectation of being able to reap in the summer; and very often, when we cannot bring something about, or prevent something, we pray, in the hope that someone else can.

Many things which happen are singular events, like an aeroplane crash; others are regular or uniform changes like the continuously changing position of the planets in their orbits around the sun. But when we ask why, we are, usually, looking for the same kind of answer in each case. We want to know what caused the event which interests us. We say: the aeroplane crashed because the pilot misread the altimeter, and as a result levelled out too soon; or that it crashed because the engine failed, causing it to lose lift. Similarly, we say that the planets move continuously in orbits around the sun because they are being pushed out by a centrifugal force and pulled in by the force of gravity, and these two forces balance each other, so causing the orbital motion. We have an unshakeable belief that, under the right conditions, one event will cause another, or what amounts to the same thing, that one event is the effect of another. We believe, that is to say, that in some cases two or more events do not happen independently of each other but are connected, and that the connexion is one of cause and effect.

And just as our dealings with other people and the objects around us exhibits the all-pervasiveness of this belief, so our language reflects it. Words like: push, pull, intervene, interfere, make, bring-about, prevent – and indeed practically all verbs – have a built-in sense of cause and effect. So, too, of course, do many nouns: if 'food' means that which nourishes and 'poison' that which harms, their meanings presuppose cause-effect relationships.

Not only this, but we have many general beliefs about causal relationships. We believe that everything which happens, every event, has a cause; and in particular that the regular patterns of changes we observe in nature always have a causal explanation. We believe that a cause, if repeated, will bring about the same effect in the same conditions; that a cause cannot occur after its effect, though it may occur at the same time; that different causes can bring about the same effect; that one cause leads to an effect which can itself be the cause of another effect; and so on. And these beliefs pay off.

Of course we sometimes get things wrong. We press the switch to make the light go on, and it fails to do so. Or we strike a match and find that it does not ignite. But such failures do not make us give up our belief in causal relationships or in any of the general principle about causation which we take for granted all the time. On the contrary, because we do believe that the same cause will produce the same effect in the same conditions, we expect the light to go on when the switch is pressed and the match to light when it is struck. So when these events fail to occur, we look for the cause of the failure. For since we also believe that every event has a cause, we take it that the non-lighting of the bulb and the match, in a context in which we expected them to light, are events which must themselves have causes. We expected something to happen which has not come about, and we ask why. So we discover that the bulb has burnt out and that the match was wet. It does not occur to us to suppose that everything is in working order and that the bulb and the match fail to light because there are no causal connexions, or because our general causal principles are incorrect. If the switch is working properly, if there is nothing wrong with the wires and they are properly connected, if the bulb is in good working order and the electricity is flowing, then the bulb *will* light. How could it fail to do so? If it does fail, there must be some reason why. There must be an intervening cause. Something has occurred which prevents the bulb from lighting.

This shows that we sometimes use one principle to bolster another even though they are independent principles. It could be true that every event has a cause yet false that the same cause will on different occasions, and under the same conditions, always produce the same effect; and it could be true that the same cause in the same conditions always produces the same effect though false that every event is caused. So these two principles are independent. Nevertheless as we have seen, the principle that every event has a cause is sometimes used to save the principle that the same cause will produce the same effect in the same conditions. For if in the past a certain cause has produced a certain effect, but when we now apply it, it fails to do so, we use the principle that every event has a cause to justify saying that the event we now have, namely the non-occurrence of an expected effect, must itself have a cause. This then enables us to say that the same cause *would have* produced the same effect *if* the conditions had been the same; if, that is, there had not been an intervening cause. Thus, we take the absence of intervening causes as a general condition which must be satisfied if *this* cause is to operate successfully. In this way we are able to retain the principle that the same cause will always produce the same effect in the same conditions, and we are able, too, to retain a belief in the particular causal relationship between, say, striking and lighting, even though there are occasions when striking is not followed by lighting.

To accept that a causal relationship continues to hold even though there are occasions when the cause does not yield the effect, is to recognise that it only holds *relatively* to certain conditions. Or, what amounts to the same thing, that certain conditions have to be satisfied before the cause can operate successfully. The match must not be wet; it must be struck in an atmosphere which contains sufficient oxygen, and so on. These are not themselves the cause of the match's lighting, for they may be present when the match does not light (because it is not struck), but they are *necessary conditions* for the successful operation of the cause in the sense that, if they are not satisfied, the match will not light even if it is struck.

The idea of a necessary condition thus provides us with a loophole defence of particular causal relationships in cases where they might seem to fail. For if our belief in a particular causal relationship is that the cause will only produce its effect provided certain necessary conditions are satisfied, it is always open to us, when a cause fails to produce its effect, to say that the conditions were not right rather than, what we would otherwise have to say, that we were wrong to think that there was a causal relationship here or that the cause has suddenly, *and for no reason*, ceased to operate. If we take a sleeping pill which fails to work, even though it has done so in the past, we can say that it may have been because there was too much alcohol in the blood, or because the blood pressure was too high, or a thousand other things, so retaining our belief in the causal relationship between taking barbiturates and falling asleep – in spite of the failure in particular cases. Of course, we cannot simply choose an arbitrary explanation of why the pill failed to work if we want the explanation to be convincing. We have to perform tests and experiments and conduct detailed investigations of the various possibilities which occur to us. But even if we fail to find a satisfactory explanation, we never give up the belief that there is one. For we never give up the belief that there must have been a cause of the failure.

Our beliefs in causal relationships, then, are not isolated beliefs about the connexion between two events of a certain kind. Since the presence of a necessary condition just is the absence of an intervening cause, or equally, the absence of a necessary condition is the presence of an intervening cause, a belief in a particular causal relationship is in fact a belief in a whole network of interconnected causal relationships.

It is interesting to see that what we identify as the cause of an event is not always a necessary condition which has to be satisfied if the event is to occur. The match may light when it is not struck – if, say, it is put into a hot oven. So striking, though the cause of lighting in particular cases, is not necessary to successful lighting because different causes can produce the same effect.

But perhaps it is wrong to identify the striking, or the putting into a hot oven, as the cause. Perhaps only in a loose sense of 'cause' can either be said to be the cause of the lighting. The real cause, it might be said, is that the match-head reaches a certain critical temperature, and that can be achieved in various ways – by friction, as in striking, or by putting into a hot oven. If we take this view, then striking the match or putting it into a hot oven are conditions which are *sufficient* to bring about the effect, provided the necessary conditions are satisfied, but they are not the immediate cause of the effect. They are in fact causes of an intermediate effect – the rise in temperature of the match-head – which is itself the real cause of the lighting; and that, the real or immediate cause, is a necessary condition. The match would not light if the temperature of the head were not raised to a certain critical level. In fact the raising of the temperature seems to be both a necessary and a sufficient condition;

for unless it is satisfied, the match will not light and if it is satisfied, that is enough for the match to light. We might then say that the immediate cause of an event just is a necessary and sufficient condition for that event to occur. But if we do say this, we ought to realise that we are not in any sense giving an explanation of what a cause is, and especially that we are not defining a cause in terms of some simpler ideas. For as we have seen, we need the idea of a cause to explain what a necessary condition is; and if we define a sufficient condition as one which is enough to bring about an effect, that is simply to define it, too, as a cause.

In any case, it is not clear that we can always characterise even an immediate cause as a necessary condition. We might say that striking that match, though not an immediate cause of the lighting, is an immediate cause of the rise in temperature. But striking is not a necessary condition for raising the temperature because putting the match into a hot oven does that too. To meet this problem in the same way as before, we then have to find an intermediate effect between striking and the rise in temperature, and perhaps there is one, but unless we are going to give up the principle that two different causes can have the same effect, or at least deny its application to immediate causes, then somewhere along the line we are going to have to say that a cause is not a necessary condition because the effect can occur without it, as the result of some other cause.

It is sometimes difficult to pick out a cause from a set of necessary conditions but we do have techniques for doing it, though they are not infallible. One test is to see if, when we prevent what we take to be the cause from occurring, the effect ceases to occur. If we drive a nail into a piece of wood by hammering and then stop hammering, the nail stops moving through the wood. But not all cases are so simple. Sometimes we cannot prevent a cause from operating – there is, for example, no way in which we can prevent the gravitational force of the sun from operating on the earth. And sometimes, though we prevent the cause, the effect may still occur even though what we took to be the cause is indeed *a* cause. If we always wash down a sleeping pill with a glass of whisky and stop taking the pill but continue taking the whisky, we might sleep just as soundly. But it might be wrong to conclude that the pill has no effect, for it might be that the pill and the whisky both separately and together induce sleep.

Another test is to vary the suspected cause and see if there are corresponding variations in the effect. If we hit the nail hard and measure how far it goes into the wood, then hit it less hard and find that it has been driven in less far, there is good reason to believe that the variation in the force of the blow has produced the variation in the distance travelled by the nail through the wood, and hence that we have discovered the right cause. If we measure the applied force and the distance travelled by the nail accurately, say by dropping different masses on the nail from the same height, we could draw up a table which correlates an amount of force with the distance travelled by the nail and so perhaps discover a functional relationship which can be expressed mathematically. We might then be able to predict that a certain force, which we have not yet tried, will drive the nail in a certain distance; and we could then check to see if we are right.

But neither of these tests adequately distinguishes causes from necessary conditions. It is characteristic of a necessary condition that a cause will not produce its effect if the condition is absent. So if we prevent the occurrence of what we take to be the cause, and the effect does not occur, we might only have discovered a necessary condition and be wrong about the cause. If a doctor gives us some simple sugar tablets and tells us that they are superb sleeping pills, it might be that every time we take one, we sleep soundly and every time we fail to take one, we spend a restless night. Yet here, it is not the pills which are causing us to sleep but the doctor's suggestion; our taking the pills is only a necessary condition. If we remove oxygen from the atmosphere, the match will not light; but the presence of oxygen is not the cause of the lighting. Similarly, if we vary the amount of oxygen, the flame burns brighter or less well, and we could discover a functional relationship between the amount of oxygen and the size and colour of the flame. But again, the amount of oxygen is not causing the match to light, though we might in this way have discovered a different causal relationship between the amount of oxygen and colour and size of the flame. In the case of the particular relationship in which we are interested, however – striking and lighting – no variation in the cause produces a variation in the effect: hard striking and gentle striking will not produce more or less lighting, either the match bursts into flame or it does not.

The beliefs we have in particular causal relationships and in general principles of causation are, then, complex and inter-related, and they are certainly not infallible; but they do work. They motivate us to find out a great deal about the world, and by and large we are successful. We want to know what causes disease, earthquakes, a rise in prices and the failure of crops, and as we find out, so we begin to understand. For one measure of understanding is control, and we are enormously successful in our control over events. In that sense, the beliefs we have and the techniques which reflect these beliefs, which we employ to investigate and discover the causes of events, pay off. But what justifies them? Is it simply the fact that they do work? That might be the answer, but if so, it seems curiously unsatisfactory. It is the punter's answer: keep backing the same horse so long as it pays off. But our beliefs are stronger than that. It is not merely that they do work, but that we cannot conceive of their failing to work. It is like having a horse which cannot lose; and that seems to call for explanation. We want to know why they work.

To refuse to ask this question, or to reply – they just do, that's all there is to it, is to put an end to rational enquiry. It is to deny in this context the naturalness and reasonableness of the very same kind of question which is so fruitful when we ask it of events themselves. We ask of particular events 'Why does that happen?', and we come up with answers about causal relationships which reveal a reliance on general principles and techniques which work. So now, when we ask 'Why do they work?', we feel that we are being fobbed off with a non-answer if we are told: they just do. Of course, in asking the question why, of the principles, we should not necessarily expect the same kind of answer that we get when we ask it of events. Whenever we ask why, we are looking for a reason or explanation, and to identify the cause of an event is to give an explanation of its occurrence. But the specification of causes is not the only kind of explanation, so we ought not to feel dissatisfied if we cannot find a causal explanation of why the causal principles work: in any case, there seems to be something circular about that. Yet it is surprising, or perhaps it is not, how hard we push for causal explanations. We might, for example, in answer to the question 'Why do the principles work?', give the answer 'Because nature is like that: natural events are connected to each other by cause-effect relations'. Yet this, too, seems to be fobbing-off, and if we feel that it is, and go on to ask why the universe or nature is so, it seems somehow more satisfying to be told, 'Because God *made* it so.'

There is even some satisfaction in saying that the principles work because *we* make them work. For there is a sense in which we do. When there is no apparent cause of an event we have a psychological need to invent one, and often do so. Suppose a window suddenly shatters. We look for a stone on the floor and a small boy in the street, and when we fail to find either, we glance at the sky to see if there is an aeroplane travelling at supersonic speed; but if there is no aeroplane, we might postulate a distant explosion which we failed to hear, or a contraction of the window frame which we failed to notice, or even, in the last resort, glass fatigue. Here we are being pushed by our principles and techniques to guess at causes which we may have no way of verifying. For the situation we have is the same, though in reverse order, as the kind of situation we construct when we seek to identify a cause by removing it. We stop hammering and the nail ceases to move; that is, we prevent the cause and so prevent the effect;

and this is what we have in the case of the shattered window, though in reverse time order. Before the window shattered, we had no cause and no effect; after it shatters, therefore, we postulate a cause. It does not occur to us to say that it shattered but there was no cause. Even if, after a long investigation we fail to discover the cause, we nevertheless believe firmly that something caused it. And if we are pressed to say why, the only answer we can give in the end is that whenever something happens, whenever there is a change of some sort, something must have caused it. Why? Because every event has a cause. Nothing happens without a cause. So we might feel inclined to say that the principles work because we make them work, or that they are true because we will not allow them to be false. Yet that kind of answer makes it look as if we invented the principles and that there is no causal order in the universe, instead we imposed one. This is not to say, of course, that we invent what happens, but rather that we invent explanations of what happens. But if the causal order is artificially imposed, then science and technology are in some sense conventional. It is not that we have discovered what is, and used it to our advantage, but that we have developed a way of looking at what happens which turns out to be of advantage. Yet if this is so, how did we get these beliefs in the first place? It surely cannot have been either a lucky accident or a deliberately invented policy.

In trying to say what justifies our belief in causal principles, or indeed in the existence of cause-effect relationships, it looks as if we have to ask how we get them. And the answer to that might seem simple. We just look around us and see what is happening. We notice that one event causes another, we notice that nothing happens without a cause, and we notice that the same cause produces the same effect. But do we?

What noticeable difference is there between one event's causing another and one event's being followed by another? If we strike a match and then it lights, we want to say that the striking caused the lighting. If we strike a match and then the telephone bell rings, we do not want to say that the striking caused the ringing. Why not? Well, because we know something about the connexion between striking and lighting, and something about the connexion between dialling and ringing, and we know that the two pairs of events are unconnected. But how do we know this? Because we know something about friction on the one hand, and telephone systems on the other; and we know that they are not connected. But this is to appeal to further causal connexions in order to explain what is now taking place. We know that friction causes a rise in temperature of the match-head, and that is why it ignites; we know that there are actual physical connexions between wires, relays and bells which explains why dialling causes ringing. So now we can ask the same question: do we notice that friction causes a rise in temperature?

If we are going to say that we get to know about causal relationships just by looking at what is going on around us, and that is what justifies our belief in them, then somewhere along the way we are going to have to say what it is that we notice which makes a causal relationship causal and what it is that is not noticeable, because it is not present, in a situation in which we want to deny a causal connexion. We can put the question off for a time by justifying a particular causal relationship (striking-lighting) in terms of another which we claim to know (friction-heating), but if, in the end, we are going to justify what we claim to know in terms of what we see, then, in the end, we have to say what we see. So what do we see in the striking-lighting (or friction-heating), and what do we fail to see in the striking-ringing?

In the case of the lighting, we see the actual physical contact of the match-head on the sandpaper. We see the head scrape across the sandpaper and burst into flame. In the case of the ringing, we see no physical contact, no contact of any sort, between the match and the sound. But that will not do. We claim to know that the relative movement of the earth and the moon causes a movement in the sea, in fact causes a regular tidal ebb and flow, but we do not see any physical contact, or contact of any sort, between the moon and the sea. Perhaps we see that as the match is scraped across the sandpaper *so* it lights. Do we? That surely is what we are trying to establish – the connexion expressed by *so*. What noticeable difference is there between events described by 'as the match is scraped across the sandpaper *so* it lights' and those described by 'the match is scraped across the sandpaper *and then* it lights'? What is the difference between the scraping's causing the lighting and the scraping's being followed by the lighting? Are we any nearer to answering this? Do we *see* a connexion which is not just temporal succession?

Perhaps we are taking 'see' or 'notice' too narrowly, or 'connexion' too strongly. It is obvious that whatever we see in causal relationships, we cannot always see a material physical connexion because there is often none there to see – there is no lump of wire connecting the moon to the sea. What we see is the movement of the moon and the movement of the water. Still, it might be said, we can *discover*, rather than see, a non-seeable, because non-material, physical 'connexion' – the force of gravity. Well, how exactly? We note down the position of the moon and the height of the tide at various times, and over a long period of time and in different parts of the world, then we 'see' that there is a connexion between the two sets of figures: that whenever the moon is in such-and-such a position relatively to the earth, the height of the water is so-and-so. We can discover a functional relationship. We can even use the tables to predict what will happen to the tides tomorrow, next week and next year. So we can; but what do we see? And what would we fail to see if it were just a chance correlation between the two sets of figures? We observe the position of the moon and the height of the tide at lots of times and in lots of places. We discover a correlation between the two sets of figures. But what justifies our saying that the movement of the moon in relation to the earth causes a change in the tide? Why, on this basis, should we not be prepared to say that the movement in the tide causes a change in the position of the moon? How do we know that there is not some external cause, which we cannot observe at all, which is causing both movements?

What is persuasive about the moon-tide situation is that there is a regularity about it. Not only is every position of the moon correlated with a position of the tide, but there is a pattern which is repeated, month after month and year after year. There are what initially appear to be irregularities – we get very high tides and very low tides at certain times of the year, but these, too, can be explained since we find that they occur when the moon is in line with the sun. We notice that the irregularities occur in a regular way and then find that they can be correlated with special events. This shows us that we also have to take into account the sun's gravitational effect on the seas, as well as the moon's, but far from disconfirming our original belief that the movement of the moon has an effect on the movement of the sea, these new facts strengthen it. Everything fits together.

So perhaps we were wrong to try to find what is characteristic of a causal connexion by looking at a singular occurrence, like the striking of a match. For even here, it is not that we have seen striking followed by lighting just once but many, many times. Lighting follows striking, not invariably, but regularly; and when it does not, we can explain the failure in terms of special circumstances, such as a damp match. By contrast, the striking of a match is only infrequently followed by the ringing of a telephone whereas dialling almost always is; and when dialling is not followed by ringing, we can explain that in terms of special circumstances – perhaps a wire is broken. Can we then say that what distinguishes a causal connexion from simple temporal succession is that, in the case of a causal connexion, the happening is of a *kind* which regularly takes place? In each particular case of the happening we do just have one event followed by another – that is all that there is to *see in* the particular occurrence; but what we can also *see about* the particular occurrence, because of our past experience, is that it is an example of a regularity.

There is no doubt that in many cases what gives rise to our belief in particular causal connexions is just that we have experienced regularities. When we see a new example of the event which comes first, we expect the second to occur, and it is natural to think that the first brings about the second. If it does not, we want to know why. We ask, what brought about the failure? Suppose, then, there are no causal *connexions* in nature, no mysterious linking force between events, but simply regular patterns of events of one kind being followed by events of another kind. It is easy to see how, in such a world, we might come to believe in the existence of causal connexions, even though there are none, and how we might come to believe general principles of the sort that every event has a cause, and that the same cause will, in the right conditions, produce the same effect. So perhaps the world is like this and there are no causal connexions. Or that might be putting it too strongly. It is not that we want to say that there are no causal connexions, but simply that causal connexions just are examples of regular happenings. That is, we have not thrown out the idea of a cause-effect relationship, but analysed it, re-expressed it, or explained what it is, in terms of something which can be observed. Previously, it seemed to be mysterious simply because we were trying to observe something special in a singular happening but could not find it. What seemed to make for a problem, then, is just that we were looking in the wrong place.

Is that all there is to it? There are after all many regularities, both natural and artificial, which no-one would dream of calling causal. A person's birth is followed by his death, regularly and inevitably, but his birth does not cause his death, though it is a necessary condition for it. Whenever the ten o'clock train leaves King's Cross for Edinburgh, the Southampton train leaves Waterloo, regularly; but the movement of one train does not cause the movement of the other.

Suppose we set two clocks going, one running five minutes behind the other. Whenever the big hand of one is at a certain point of its dial, the big hand of the other is at a point five minutes ahead on its dial. Here is a regularity. We can draw up a table which correlates the positions of the two hands and use it to predict occurrences which have not yet taken place. We can say that when the first clock reads 9.06, the second will read 9.11; and when the time comes we can check to see if we were right. Does the movement of one hand cause the movement of the other? But why not? What is the difference between this and the moon-tide situation? Just the artificiality of the one and the naturalness of the other? But suppose the movements of the moon and the sea are both caused by some third external force but are not otherwise related. The clocks might be like that; they might both be electric clocks running from the same power source.

We might say that we can stop the first clock and the second would not stop, but if we could stop the relative movement of the moon and the earth, the sea would cease to ebb and flow. But how do we know this if the only thing we have to go on is the regularity? We certainly cannot put it to the test by stopping the moon from moving relatively to the earth. It may be that in some cases we can distinguish artificial or accidental regularities from those which we want to call causal by applying this kind of test. For we might expect that in the genuinely causal case, the effect will cease if the cause ceases, whereas in the non-causal case, the cessation of one event will not be followed by a cessation in the other. If this is so, however, an explanation of causal connexions cannot be given in terms of simple regularity alone. Instead, we have to say something like: an event followed by another is a case of a causal connexion if the happening is an example of a regular succession and is such that if an event of the first kind does not occur, an event of the second kind does not occur. But as we have seen, this is not strong enough; for the absence of one event followed by the absence of the other is not adequate in distinguishing causes from necessary conditions. If we prevent a birth we prevent a death. And even if we build more tests into the criterion, by saying, for example, that a variation in an event of the first kind must be followed by a variation in an event of the second kind, still we shall not have an adequate means of distinguishing regular successions which can be identified as causal from those which cannot.

So how do we distinguish causal regularities from others? The trouble is, the only kind of answer which seems to be at all satisfying is that a non-accidental regularity is *the result of* a causal relationship. We want to say that events of one kind are regularly followed by events of a second kind in a non-accidental way when events of the first kind *cause* events of the second kind, or when both are caused by something else. We can explain regularities, and the differences between different kinds of regularities, in terms of causes but not, it seems, the other way round.

Yet if it is true that we might come to believe in causal relationships as a result of noticing regularities, and if it is true, as it seems to be, that we can to some extent control our environment by noticing and taking advantage of the fact that one kind of event is regularly followed by another, without ever asking why, or perhaps, if we ask why, without its making any difference what answer we give, what do we gain by supposing that there is something more? If the only evidence we have is the observation of regularities, and if we have tests which do enable us in some cases to discriminate them, what advantage is there in describing some regularities as causal?

For even if we are right, and they are causal, we do not gain any further insight. Causal or not, in our dealings with them we are still limited by the evidence we have; that is, by the observation of regular sequences and the results of the tests. The tests are not infallible, but they are generally useful; and because that is all we have to go on whether or not there are causal connexions, we do not need to postulate connexions. We notice the regularities and we apply the tests whenever we can. In this way we gain control over our environment. So perhaps we do not need to know why something happens; perhaps it is enough just to know that it does. Perhaps when we say this happened *because* that happened, we are not saying anything which is more useful and informative than: this happened and then that happened. If we put a magnet near enough to some iron filings, we see the iron filings move towards the magnet; if we put a block of wood between the magnet and the filings, we see they cease to move. And we can use these facts to our advantage. What does it add to our knowledge, or to our ability to control events, if we ask why, and come up with the answer that the filings are attracted by a magnetic force and that placing a piece of wood in the right place can be used as an intervening cause to prevent the force from operating? If the world just is like that – there are regularities and there is no more to it – we shall be no worse off. Anything more, any explanation we might give, is theory not fact.

Why does this way of looking at things seem so unsatisfactory? For one thing, it puts a limit to rational enquiry in that it makes asking why a pointless exercise. And it does violence to the way we do conduct our enquiries. The observation of naturally occurring regularities is important because it is the starting place for most investigations, but it is only a starting place. By contrast, the attempt to answer the question why leads to new discoveries and technologies. Perhaps it is just theory and not fact that there is a magnetic force, but if it were not for the theory, who would have thought of rotating a magnet inside a wire coil in order to produce electricity? There were no naturally occurring regularities to be observed here; instead, new situations and new regularities were *created* because of the belief in a magnetic force. And if it is just theory, with no factual content, it is surprising, in fact incredible, that it led to new discoveries.

If a farmer has two fields in one of which the crops always flourish and in the other always fail, whatever he plants, he can notice a regularity; and he can learn from it and take advantage of it. He can cut his losses and refrain from planting seeds in the bad field. But it is doubtful if the regularity of itself would ever lead him to discover that the bad field had a serious nitrogen deficiency. He, or someone, has to ask why; he has to discover what is causing the failure of the crops and come up with the *right* answer. Then he can put the field right.

More important, however, is the fact that an account of causation in terms of regularities denies the very possibility of unique causal happenings. Yet there seems to be nothing absurd in the idea that an event causes another once and once only. Imagine a world in which there is just one combustible object. On a very hot day, it bursts into flame. The event can never be repeated because there is nothing else which will burn, but is it absurd to say that the object burst into flame because the sun heated it to a critical temperature? It might be said that we, from the point of view of our world, can see this as a causal happening because we are familiar with events of that *kind*. We already know of regularities into which it fits. But the inhabitants of that world, incombustible as they are, would not be able to see this as a causal event. Then what are they to say of it, that it is uncaused? In any case, what they or we would say is beside the point. The point is whether it *is* a non-causal sequence just because it is not an example of a regular sequence. Imagine a world in which there are no regularities at all. One day lightning is followed by thunder, on another by rain, on another by clear weather; and so for all events. Does it make no sense to say that in such a world some events cause others? Or are we to say that every event is uncaused? What would an uncaused event be like? It would happen spontaneously and come from nothing.

There is a sense in which we might say that an uncaused event happens by chance, but this cannot be the sense of 'chance' which we normally have in mind when we describe, say, the behaviour of a roulette ball. When we say that the roulette ball falls into zero by chance, because it might have fallen into many other slots, we do not mean that the event was uncaused. We mean, rather, that the causal explanation is so complicated that we are not in a position to give it, but if we knew all the factors – the force applied to the wheel and the ball, the amount of friction, the starting position of the wheel and the ball, and so on – we could work out the path of the ball and know which slot it would fall in. We say that it fell into zero by chance because, from the point of view of our knowledge, it might as well be uncaused, not because we believe it to be uncaused. Or we can say that the probability of its falling into zero is, given a fair wheel, but the probability of an event is a measure of our ignorance about causes, not a characteristic feature of an uncaused event.

It is not simply that we can imagine worlds in which singular causal events occur, but that we often take them to occur in our world. Just this genetic heritage and this set of environmental conditions produced this man; in consequence he has unique physical features and a unique personality which are characteristic of him and him alone. There are, of course, numerous and complex regularities involved in this, but the total set of circumstances which constitute the cause is unique and the effect is unique. If it were not so, we should not be able to identify a criminal by his fingerprints. Similarly, though there have been many aeroplane crashes, and though the causes have been similar in some cases and many regularities are involved in the assessment of the cause of any particular one, the set of circumstances associated with each crash is unique. But this does not prevent our discovering what the particular cause is, nor does it deter us from apportioning blame and punishment on the basis of the assessment. Or again, what a husband says to his wife on a particular occasion may cause her great distress, though it would not have the same effect on her in different circumstances or on others in any circumstances; yet it is what he says on that occasion which causes her distress.

Natural regularities are important as a basis for science, but only as a basis; and they are an important factor in a psychological account of how we come to believe in causes, but only a factor. In neither case do they seem to be necessary. For it seems reasonable to suppose that the caveman who first used a lever had not observed any appropriate regularities in nature. He might have been playing idly with a piece of wood, holding one end in his hand while the middle rested on a stone. Still playing, he pushed the other end under another stone and pressed down with his hand. Would he not *see*, immediately, that pushing his hand down made the other end come up and lift the second stone? Could he not discover a causal relationship in the one case? He might then go on to experiment, using different amounts of pressure and different sized stones, and so make regular sequences occur because he knows the causal relations which can be used to make them. And he could develop a theory about them in terms of the amount of force applied at certain distances from the pivot and the masses which could be lifted. So he could get a knowledge of causal relationships, and begin to construct a science, independently of observing regularities, though he could use the causal relationsip to *produce* regularities – every time a certain force is used, a certain mass can be lifted. Then, perhaps, when he later notices regularities occurring in nature, he might reasonably wonder what causes them. That, surely, is why we want to say that regularities may be the result of causal relationships but do not in any way explain them. We could of course describe this situation by saying that he pushed down with a certain force *and then* a mass of a certain size was lifted. But the reason why we want to say that this is an inadequate account is simply that one event follows the other, in this case, only because it is caused by the other. If it were not caused, it would not follow. In any case, the analysis has to go further than that. If the whole explanation of causation is going to be in terms of temporal succession, we cannot say that he *pushed* down, or that the mass was *lifted*. We have to say: his arms moved, the wood moved, the stone moved; and that is all.

Yet if we want to say that there is more to it than this, we have to say what it is that the caveman sees, when he spots the causal connexion between pressing the wood and lifting the stone, that he would not see in the case of a non-causal correlation. Perhaps he does *see that* there is a causal connexion, but is this because he actually sees the connexion? Well, it is one bit of wood he has, so he can *see* the physical connexion between the two ends; and because of this he can *see that* if he moves the wood at all, he moves both ends of it. To move one end is to move the wood, and that is to move the other end. If we pull one end of a piece of string, we see the other end move; so we see that pulling one end *makes* the other end move, because we see both ends as part of the same bit. And when one end of the lever is moved and a stone rests on the other end, we see that this makes the stone move just because we have, as it were, joined the wood and the stone and made one thing out of them. This, too, is something we see. When we couple a truck to an engine and the engine moves, we see the hook on the engine bang against the ring of the truck, we see the truck jerk and move; and so we *see that* the movement of the engine causes the movement in the truck because, having coupled the two together, that is really no different from seeing one thing move. But seeing one thing move is not seeing one event followed by, or contemporaneous with, another. It is seeing one event. And we do not need regular sequences to see it. We just need the one event. After that, we can construct regular sequences. We make engines for the purpose of pulling trucks.

But of course not all causal connexions can be explained in terms of physical connexions – we still have the problem of the moon and the tides. Here we cannot see any sort of connexion. Yet if we can see causal connexions in some cases, and produce regularities by manipulating causes, it is certainly not irrational to postulate them in other cases where we cannot see them, provided there is some kind of evidence, such as observed regular sequences, which suggests that there is a causal connexion there. Of course we might be wrong when we generalise in this way, but there is no reason to suppose that we are wrong *in principle* in cases where we can only observe the regularity and not the connexion.

We often generalise on the basis of observable evidence to the existence of something which cannot be observed. We believe with good reason that there are colours which we cannot see and sounds which we cannot hear. Dogs react when we blow a Galton whistle which makes no sound to us, their ears regularly prick up when we blow and fall flat when we stop blowing. And that is very good evidence both that there is a sound and that it is causing the dog to prick up its ears. But because in this case we cannot perceive directly either the cause or the connexion, such as the sound waves impinging on the ear drum, we ought to be less sure of ourselves; we might be wrong. And in general, we cannot expect every regular sequence to be the result of a causal connexion when the connexion itself cannot be perceived. For the fact that causal connexions can be used to bring about regular sequences is not enough to tell us that every regular sequence is brought about in this way. But if we apply to regularities all the tests which in general seem to characterise those causal relationships in which we can see the connexion – if we remove or vary what we take to be the cause and find that the effect ceases or varies – then we have a better chance of being right. Still we might be wrong because the tests are not decisive, but that is a risk we always take when we rely on evidence for what is rather than direct observation of what is. That we might sometimes be wrong, however, is not to say that we cannot ever be right, or that we are wrong to suppose there is more to some regularities than the regularity.

In a sense, *any* two events can be taken to be an example of a bizarre regularity. When the train moves, the Tower of London stays where it is, regularly; and when the train stands still, the Tower stays where it is, regularly. But it would be absurd to say that the train's movement causes the Tower to stay where it is, or that its standing still also causes it to stay where it is, or that whatever the train does, it causes the Tower to remain by the Thames. And it would be absurd just because whatever we do to the supposed cause, whether we prevent it or vary it, nothing happens to the effect. But why, after all, are such tests good working principles which do discriminate some regularities from others if in *all* cases there is just the regularity and no further connexion?

Chapter 2

NATURAL LAWS

Will the future be like the past? Not in every respect, of course; there may never be another war; we may one day have world government; people change their minds and adopt different behaviour patterns; next year there may be an unusually cold summer and a very warm winter; people, plants and animals now alive will eventually die; and so on. Even things which happen habitually might one day be different. Certain species of birds always build nests, but we can imagine a gradual evolutionary change leading to a future in which they no longer do so. The planets follow their predictable orbits around the sun but there might be a cataclysmic astronomical event, such as the explosion of the sun, which would end that. In fact, when we take into account all the changes which we can imagine or might expect to take place, it seems a funny question to ask. Yet there are things which we believe have always happened in the past, which happen now, and which always will happen. Metals always expand when heated; a solid lump of lead never floats on water, but ice and oil always do; a heavy object dropped from a height always falls to the ground. Could such things change?

Of course, even these beliefs are hedged about with conditions. We do not believe that in every conceivable set of circumstances a heavy object will always fall to the ground when dropped from a height: if it is a piece of iron and there is a very powerful magnet suspended above it, it will move up, not down. Cream always floats on milk, but ingenious tinkerers with natural processes have managed to create homogenised milk in which it does not. We often know how to prevent the operation of natural processes, but we still believe they are continuing to operate, undercover as it were, and that we need actively to suppress or counter them if we want to avoid their effects. The way we suppress them, however, is by taking advantage of other natural processes. It is only because a sufficiently powerful magnet will always attract a piece of iron of an appropriate size that we can use the force of magnetism to counter the force of gravity. We can make metal ships which float and metal aeroplanes which fly, not because metal has suddenly ceased to sink in water or to fall to the ground when released from a height, but because a sufficiently

large box of air will always float and because even a heavy object
which has enough forward motion relatively to the air will always
have enough lift to prevent its falling. Natural processes can be
played off one against another to achieve a desired outcome, but if
they were not in some sense continuing all the time, this playing-off
technique would not work. That tomorrow a solid lump of iron will
float and a large box of air will sink, is a future we do not con-
template.

These naturally occurring regularities, which often make us
suspect a causal relationship, reflect what we sometimes call natural
laws, or laws of nature. We believe in a uniformity of natural processes which reveal themselves as regularities under the right conditions – which usually means under natural conditions, or conditions
which we have not interfered with. And even if there are no further
revealed regularities, we still believe that the laws hold good. It may
be that no-one will ever again put a solid lump of metal into water,
but what we believe, without question, is that if someone *were* to do
so, though in fact he does not, it *would* sink. That is what a belief
in a natural law is. It is a belief which is to some extent independent
of what actually happens; and it is a belief which embraces the past,
the present and the future. This is why we believe the future will be
like the past in many important respects.

But what justifies such a belief? We might say that natural
regularities are the result of causal relationships, and because we can,
if we are tough-minded enough, justify our beliefs in causal relationships by holding that we sometimes perceive causal connexions, so
it might be claimed that we have a well-grounded belief in natural
laws. But that is not good enough. For even if we can perceive some
causal connexions, we rarely if ever perceive those which give rise
to natural regularities. We see the rock sink, but we do not see what
makes it sink. We can heat a piece of iron and see it expand, and we
might claim to perceive the cause of the expansion, namely the
application of heat; even so, we do not see the heat making the metal
expand. We do not, that is to say, perceive the causal connexion.
We have a regularity which makes us suspect such a connexion, but
when we infer to the belief that there is one, we have to acknowledge
that we may be wrong to do so. And this is so even if the standard
tests work – we stop heating and the expansion stops, or we vary the
amount of heat and notice a variation in the amount of expansion.
None of these things are decisive. And in cases where we cannot
perceive either the cause or the connexion, such as the operation of
the force of gravity, the inference we make receives only slender
support from an analogy with those cases, like the operation of a
lever, in which we might claim to see both.

But there is more to it than this. For even if we could in all cases perceive both the cause and the connexion, could we see also that it will always work in just the way it is now doing? How could we see the future in the observation of what is? We might say we can see that the application of this kind of cause *must* produce this kind of effect, and if we can see what must be so, we can see what will be so; for what must be, will be. Yet how could we, in seeing the connexion, see also that it could not possibly be otherwise? How could we see, not just the connexion, but that it is in some sense necessary or inevitable; that it must always be as it now is? What feature does it have which shows us that it must be so? In any case, if in some situations, perhaps all, we do not see connexions, then in those situations we do not see necessary connexions.

We may well feel that we can justify a general belief in the existence of causal relationships by claiming that we can sometimes perceive causal connexions – and that might be a very strong claim. But we obviously cannot claim that every particular belief in the existence of particular causal relationships can be justified in this way. Where we have to acknowledge that we cannot perceive either the cause or the connexion, the justification has to be different. We have to say, perhaps, that since in those cases where we can perceive the connexion, we can often manipulate the cause to produce a regularity, so, when we perceive a natural regularity, we have good reason to suspect a causal connexion. Perhaps we are right when we make such a guess, though we could be wrong. But even if we were always right, there is still nothing to tell us that connexions which have operated in the past will always continue to do so in the future. For even where we might claim to see connexions, we can scarcely claim to see in them that they will always operate as they now do. To justify a general belief in causal connexions, then, is still a long way from justifying a belief in natural laws. To justify the latter is essentially to justify the general principle that the same cause will, under the same conditions, *always* produce the same effect. That seems difficult enough. But it is even worse if we take the view that there are no causal connexions, for then, the belief that natural regularities will continue in the future as they have in the past has to be justified in terms of the regularities themselves, and that is impossible.

When we say that metals expand when heated, we not only refer to past and present cases which have been observed, and project these to the future, we project also to the past and present. We believe that on innumerable occasions in the past metals have expanded when heated, by the sun perhaps, even though no-one observed what was happening; that they are expanding now as a result of heat, in places where there is no-one to see; and that they will expand under the influence of heat in the future even though there is no-one left alive to see what is taking place. Yet our only evidence for this seems to be that on some occasions in the past and present, some examples of this regularity have been observed. If this is so, however, our beliefs reach out far beyond the evidence we have.

But perhaps the evidence is better than that. For at least, so far as the future is concerned, we have in the past held similar beliefs about what was then the future and these turned out to be justified when that future was realised. Futures which have now gone by did resemble the past, and that seems to be evidence that the future is always like the past. But is there anything in this to tell us that the future we have not yet experienced is going to be like the past? We seem here simply to be trading on the assumption that what was, will be. The fact that three days ago we expected metals to expand when heated today, and that this expectation has been justified, tells us nothing about tomorrow unless we assume that past uniformities will continue. But that is just the assumption at issue. In any case, even if the fact that futures now gone by did resemble the past were to give us some feeling of security about tomorrow, it does nothing whatever to justify a projection to past events which have not been observed. For we cannot go back to see whether that assumption pays off.

Are our beliefs really as strong as that? Do we really believe that there never will be, or never could be, a day on which a solid lump of lead floats on water? Well, if it really is ordinary lead and ordinary water and no tinkering has taken place – we have not slipped a bit of transparent plastic beneath the lead or otherwise introduced intervening causes – then, yes, that is what we believe. But suppose the structure of lead changes radically so that its density becomes much less than that of water. Is such a change impossible? Perhaps not; but would it then be an ordinary bit of lead? Surely some tinkering has taken place here, not by us but by nature, and there will be a causal explanation of it, though we might never be able to discover what it is. If such a thing happened, we might well choose to call this 'new-lead' and say that it resembles the old lead, which no longer exists, in all respects other than the change in structure and density. Then we could still say of the old lead that if there were any, though there is not, and if it were put in water, though it cannot be, it would sink. But that makes it look as if natural laws are true of the future because we will not let them be otherwise. When we get a massive failure, we do not count it as a failure.

What exactly are our beliefs? We certainly believe that lead, the stuff we now have, will always sink in water. But we surely do not mean to deny the very possibility of a future change in the structure of lead. After all, we can envisage such changes and conceive of possible explanations, such as the long-term effect of cosmic rays or some other natural phenomenon. Suppose, then, we put a bit of lead into water and it floats. We can invoke the principle that the same cause will under the right conditions always produce the same effect, to justify the conclusion that one of the necessary conditions has not been satisfied; and we might say that if it were satisfied, lead would still sink. But that is only a first step; and if we simply stopped there, we should not have a very useful or interesting science. Normally, however, we should go on to ask which condition had failed. If we then discovered that the structure of lead had changed, we might indeed describe this fact by saying that we now have new-lead. But that, too, would not be very useful or interesting. Since one of the conditions has failed, and we know which one, we can now invoke the principle that every event has a cause and ask why this particular change took place.

This procedure is rational because it is a technique which relates past knowledge to new and unexpected events. Faced by the un-expected events, we could simply say that the old law 'Lead sinks in water' is now false, and so dismiss it from further consideration; or we could say that it remains true but there is no longer any lead about, and so make the law inapplicable and useless. But each of these attitudes puts an end to enquiry because each ignores the essential fact that some change has taken place which *relates* the past sinking of lead to its present floating. To take this fact into account, however, is to recognise that though the old law cannot remain as it is, it cannot simply be rejected either, for that would be to discard what knowledge we have of the past. Instead, it has to be modified, and in such a way that it accounts both for known past happenings and for what is now taking place. It remains true that lead did sink; it is true that now it does not. What we must seek to do, therefore, is to relate these two truths in one new all-embracing law. In this way we get new knowledge. Our past beliefs and present happenings *together* motivate new enquiries and lead to new discoveries.

Imagine people who have discovered that water boils at 100°C and who believe that it does so everywhere. If their travellings keep them near enough to sea level, this belief will serve them well enough. Such minor discrepancies as they might discover in their readings could be put down to calibration errors in their thermo-meters. But if, one day, they travel to the top of a mountain, they will find that all their thermometers are reading low. They must now ask why. They cannot simply accept the new event and say that water does not boil at 100°C. For it has always done so in the past, and if they go down to sea level again they will find that it still does so. They have discovered that being at sea level is a necessary condition for water to boil at 100°C and they must ask why. So they might come to discover that air pressure is an important factor in the boiling point of water.

What does this amount to? Are we now saying that our beliefs in natural laws are not really as strong as we normally suppose but rather, that they are more like hypotheses or assumptions which we take to be true until they let us down – knowing that, if they do let us down, we can handle the situation? Well, perhaps; and another way of describing it might be to say that our attitude to natural laws, as reflected by our techniques of enquiry, is much more like our attitude to habitual or dependent regularities than we might initially have expected. We certainly believe that the planets will be orbiting the sun tomorrow, next week, next year and in a thousand years, but we do not believe it to be inevitable. On the contrary, there is good reason to believe that the sun's mass will eventually change sufficiently to bring about a change in the effect of its gravitational field. Even if this were not so, we can imagine other things which might happen to destroy or change radically the movement of the planets. And perhaps the only difference between this and the belief that lead always sinks in water is that there is *at present* no good reason to suppose that lead will not always sink and it is, besides, difficult to imagine extraordinary changes which would make it float. So we might say that the difference we feel in our beliefs about natural laws and habitual regularities is one of degree, not of kind; and that this is so because there is really no difference in kind between what we choose to call law-like relationships and those we call habitual or dependent.

To take this view is as good as to say that we do not in fact believe, and certainly do not know, that the future will be like the past. We only act as if it will be. And this behaviour is justified because, when any particular expectation lets us down, we can always find an explanation and modify appropriately the particular law which gave rise to it. What a belief in laws of nature really amounts to is a belief in the permanent possibility of explanation when things go wrong, and it is a belief which is justified by the techniques we use. It is a belief in method, and the method works. But it is not simply the fact that the method does work which justifies the belief; it is, rather, the fact that we can see why it works. For the future has never really been like the past at all.

What we take to be natural laws are always failing. That aeroplanes do not, usually, fall to the ground *does* refute the law that heavy objects always fall to the ground. But here the reason for the failure is now so obvious that we do not even bother to write in the modification 'provided they do not have enough relative forward motion to create lift'. In any case, natural laws would become impossibly complex if we wrote in explicitly all the necessary conditions. So when aeroplanes do not fall to the ground, we do not reckon this as a failure in the law, instead we see it immediately as the failure of an implicit necessary condition. Sometimes, however, if the reason for the failure is not obvious, the explanation may be more complicated and the law may have to be modified explicitly. But whenever failures of any kind occur, our techniques of enquiry demand that we look for a connexion between what was and what is. These techniques ensure, therefore, that any new law explains both those past events which led us to a belief in the old law and the new unexpected events which now make us question it. In this way *we* relate the past to the present by the way we explain the differences. But the present was the future; and in what is now the future, we can do the same thing. Since we adopt as a working principle the belief that every event has a cause, we are compelled by our technique to look for the cause when a law fails; and in the last resort, if we cannot find one we can always, at least for a time, invent one. We can then say that the earlier law failed because we did not know enough about nature and had insufficient evidence on which to base it. And when we find an explanation which seems adequately to account for all the facts, past and present, we can say that we have uncovered yet another of nature's mysteries. But then, when we have the new law which explains both our past and present evidence, we act as if, and perhaps believe, that it is unassailable. And this is sensible so long as it does not let us down. If it does let us down, and no doubt it will, we know what to do.

But it cannot be as simple as that. To interpret an unexpected event as the failure of a particular law, and to explain it by modifying the law appropriately, always presupposes that other laws do not fail. No one law can ever be tested in isolation, for in the testing of it we rely on the fact that other laws are not in doubt. When we test the boiling point of water with a thermometer, we take for granted the law that metals expand when heated, and indeed that a particular amount of heat always produces a particular amount of expansion. Otherwise, we could not take the reading of the mercury as indicating anything. So when we find that all our thermometers read low if immersed in boiling water at the top of a mountain, this may be indicative of a failure in the law that mercury expands by a given amount when a certain amount of heat is applied to it. Or we might say we have a choice between that law and the law that water always boils at 100°C. And it would seem to be just as rational, or at least just as consistent with our techniques, to conclude that air pressure affects the expansion of mercury rather than, what we do conclude, that pressure affects the boiling point of water. If lead floats, it may be because the density of water has changed rather than the density of lead.

Of course in such cases there are other tests we can make. We can boil other liquids at altitude, use other metals, test the expansion of mercury by applying known amounts of heat directly to it, and so on. But in all such tests, when we put one law in doubt, we can only do so by relying on the invariance of others. We test the coherence of a bundle of laws and we are faced with making some modification to the bundle when an unexpected set of events takes place, but in the end, any *explanation* of the change which results in the modification of a particular law is only as good as the degree of reliance we put on the rest. When we measure the size of a room, we take it for granted that our measuring rod does not expand or contract at room temperatures, that the room itself will not differ in size in different conditions, and so on. But it is what we take for granted that reveals our beliefs in natural laws. This is so whether we are performing a simple operation like measuring a room or conducting a complex scientific experiment. If, during the course of an experiment, and as a minor part of it, a scientist takes the temperature of some water, and the result of the experiment throws doubt on some law, it only does so on the implicit assumption that metals always expand by a certain amount when heated by a certain amount. We can only doubt something against a presumed stable background. It is only if there are some constancies that change is explicable. We can always explain the failure of particular laws, but only given others which do not fail.

Perhaps a belief in laws of nature does not amount to any more than a belief in the permanent possibility of explanation, but such a possibility presupposes an account of change in terms of constancy. Our belief in laws of nature is at least a belief in relative constancy, a belief in coherence, and a belief that not everything could go wrong overnight. For if everything did go wrong overnight, our techniques of enquiry would cease to have value; they could not succeed.

We cannot, then, account for our belief that the future will be like the past by claiming that it is really only a belief in the effectiveness of our methods and that these work because, in a sense, we make them work. For they will cease to work, however ingeniously we apply them, unless the future does resemble the past in some respects.

Chapter 3

PERCEPTION

What would it take to convince someone that there is a brown piano in the next room, that it is smooth and shiny, is made of wood, smells of polish and makes rather a harsh jangling noise when it is played? We could tell him, but he might not believe us. But if we take him into the next room and show him, he could not fail to be convinced. He could see that it is brown and shiny; he could rub his fingers along it and feel that it is smooth; he could probably feel, as well as see, that it is made of wood; he could smell the polish, he could press a few keys and hear the noise; and he could relate all these things to his past experience and recognise that it is a piano. And because he not only sees it but feels it, smells it and hears it, he knows there really is a piano there and that it is not some clever optical illusion concocted with lights and mirrors. If it were just an optical illusion, however convincingly done, he would be able to see it but he could not rub his hands over it, play it and smell it. That it is a real piano is confirmed by the fact that his different senses corroborate each other in the way we expect them to when dealing with real objects. Seeing, touching, hearing, smelling and tasting, is the most direct evidence, and usually the only evidence, we ever have or ever could have for the belief that there are objects in the world besides ourselves and that they have certain features. Perceiving is believing.

But what exactly do we believe? When we are convinced by what we have perceived that there is a piano in the next room, we ascribe to it an independent existence, a life of its own as a solid, continuing object. We accept that it would still be there even if we were to walk out of the room and no longer see it; and we believe that when there is no-one in the room to see it, it nevertheless has the same shape, size, smell and colour which we perceive it to have when we are in the room. For when we see the size, shape and colour, or when we smell it, or try to lift it and feel the weight, we take it that these are features of *it*, that in a funny sense of 'belong' they belong to it and make it what it is. We say that *the piano* is brown, rectangular, smells of polish and weighs half a ton. And so we usually take it that if someone else were now to walk into the room, he would see exactly what we see, hear what we hear when the keys are struck, feel what we feel when we rub our fingers over it, and smell the polish as we do. For he is perceiving the piano and the piano has these features.

And yet, if this is what we believe, then our beliefs outstrip the evidence. Suppose we were in the room five minutes ago looking at the piano and that we are now outside the room. No-one else has entered and no-one else is in the room. Why does the perceptual experience which we had five minutes ago justify the belief that the piano *now* has just those features which we perceived it to have, or even that there is a piano there at all? We cannot look to check; for if we look, we are perceiving it at the time of looking, not at the time at which it was not being perceived. We might say that if we now go into the room and have the same sort of experience as we had five minutes ago, we have good evidence that it remained the same throughout the five minutes. But why? Perhaps we have perceived the piano many, many times and on each occasion it was the same; even so, our evidence is still fragmentary. Certainly the uniformity of our experiences may well bring about the belief that the piano is always as it is now perceived to be, but still we do not have and could not have direct evidence of how it is when it is not being perceived. And when we do perceive it, do we perceive that it has an independent continuing existence? Is that like perceiving its colour? Or is it rather that we ascribe an independent continuing existence to it in order to make sense of, or link together, our fragmentary but uniform experiences? Is the belief in independent continuously existing objects, and the belief that they have features when they are not being perceived which are like their perceived features, part of a commonsense *theory* about the world which imposes a coherence on our experiences? There are really two questions here: do objects exist when we are not perceiving them and, if they do, do they have the features which we commonly ascribe to them? But there is a question which comes before each of these: do objects have the features which we commonly ascribe to them even when we are perceiving them?

Is *the piano* brown? Some people are colour blind and do not see what we see. They may describe what they see as we do, having learnt to talk as we do, but there are tests we can give them which will show that they do not see colours as we do. But that, it might be said, is a defect in them and has nothing to do with the fact that the piano is brown. It *is* brown, but they see it *as* grey; and we can say this, rather than that it is grey and *we* see it as brown, because we know that they have abnormal vision which can be explained and related to ours and to the colour of the piano. Then suppose some-one with normal vision sees the piano in a very dim light, or when illuminated by a strong blue light; he will not see that it is brown.

It could be replied to this that these things, too, are explicable; indeed the very way in which they are described indicates that the conditions for seeing are not standard. Yet that makes it look as if, when we say the piano is brown, we mean only that someone with normal vision and in normal conditions will see it *as* brown; but if this is so, can we really say that the colour is a feature of the piano? It seems, rather, as if its colour is in some sense a conventional feature of it rather than an actual feature. For when we say that it *has* a particular colour, we are only saying how it will appear in certain conventional conditions. Perhaps the most we ought to say is that it has some colour or other, but depending on the conditions of illumination and the observer so it will appear differently to different people, or to the same person under different conditions. But we were taking it, initially, that we see it as it *is*; that it really is as it appears to be. And there seems, after all, to be a real difference between a green piano and a red piano which can only be accounted for by the fact that *they* have different colours, whatever variations they might be seen to have by different people. Yet if our evidence is what we see, and if that is going to be different for different people, how can we say what colour the pianos have? A green piano may look like a red piano under the right kind of illumination, even to a normal observer. Nor can we say that they will always look different if they are illuminated in the same way; for a person who is red-green blind will see them both as the same shade of grey under the same illumination. What justifies the inference from 'Charlie sees a red piano' to 'The piano is red'? And is there any difference between that, and the inference from 'Most of us see a red piano' to 'The piano is red'? The weight of numbers increases the amount of evidence, perhaps, but does it make a difference to the kind of evidence?

When we say that the piano is shiny, we surely do not mean to say that the shininess is a feature of the piano. We all know that the amount of light and the direction from which it is coming are crucial here. Could it even be sensibly said that the piano is shiny in the dark? So why do we think it sensible to say that it has a colour in the dark – and not merely *a* colour, but a particular colour? How could we possibly justify the inference from 'Most of us see a red piano under normal daylight conditions' to 'The piano is red in the dark'? There is an inference here because nobody sees it as red, or any other colour, in the dark. So what do we mean when we say that the piano is red in the dark – that if a normal observer were to switch on a normal white light, he would see it as red? But that only tells us *what would happen if*, how could it tell us *what is*?

One way out of all this would be to provide an explanation which links the different facts together. Suppose we say that every object has some feature which somehow causes observers to see particular colours under certain conditions. What we describe as seeing a colour could then be considered as the effect of a complicated causal relationship. The object provides some input to the total effect but so does the observer, since if his eyes and nervous system were different he would see differently, and so do the conditions under which the observation takes place. This sort of account would enable us to explain why, if the conditions are varied, the seen-colour is different, and also why the seen-colour might be different if the observer is different.

Just this kind of explanation is provided by the standard scientific theory of colour perception. When light strikes the surface of an object, some of it is absorbed and some is reflected. The mixture of wavelengths which is reflected depends partly on the original mixture of wavelengths in the incident light and partly on the molecular structure of the surface. The reflected light then strikes the eye and triggers off electro-chemical processes in the optic nerves which in turn stimulate the visual area of the brain and cause us to see. For us to see a particular colour, the colour receptors in the eye, the cones, have to be stimulated by a certain proportional mixture of wavelengths; and since this mixture will depend on the nature of the incident light and on the nature of the surface, both the kind of illumination and the kind of surface will play a part in determining what colour we see. But so, too, will our nervous systems; for if someone has defective cones, he will not see the colour we see even though the same reflected light strikes his eye. So we have a general causal theory of colour perception which explains why most of us would see a particular object as red in ordinary daylight, why some of us would not, and why none of us would under unusual lighting conditions. The theory carries conviction because of its general explanatory power, since both normal and abnormal visual experiences are linked together and explained in the same kind of way, and because it enables us to predict the particular colour a person will see in particular conditions.

But now what does it mean to say that *the piano* is red? In terms of the theory, if we take 'The piano is red' to be describing a feature of the piano, rather than the effect which we experience when we look at the piano, it can only be a remark about the particular molecular structure of the surface which can be correlated with various effects in various conditions. It is that physical feature of the piano which can be correlated with a normal observer's seeing red in normal daylight, an abnormal observer's seeing grey, say, in normal daylight, a normal observer's seeing green in other conditions of illumination, and so on. But a molecular structure is not a colour. Nor could it even be sensibly said that the molecular structure is coloured. Since the theory explains colour perception as an effect produced by certain causal factors, there is no place in it, nor could there be, for the ascription of colour to one of those factors. We might say, perhaps, that the theory explains what it is for the piano *to be* red, but that can only be shorthand for saying that it explains what it is for the piano to be perceived as red. The point of the theory is to explain colour perception, and part of the explanation is that one of the necessary conditions for a certain kind of colour perception to occur is the presence of a certain kind of molecular surface structure. But the kind of structure cannot itself be characterised in terms of colour, otherwise we should have no explanation at all. If the theory is correct, it cannot make sense to say that the piano *has* the colour which most of us see it to have, that it has a colour in the dark, or even that it has a colour at all, if by such remarks we mean that it, the piano, really is coloured. But if the theory is not correct, how are we to explain the different perceptions of different people under the same conditions, or of the same people under different conditions?

It is not only colour which presents a problem. If we take what appears to be a straight stick and immerse half of it in water, leaving half projecting above the surface, it appears to be bent where it meets the water. When we take it out of the water, it appears to be straight. If we put on spectacles of a certain kind, it appears to be curved. Is the stick straight, bent or curved? Shape, too, as well as colour, seems to depend on the conditions under which the observation is made – and on the observer, for there may well be people with defective vision who always see what we call straight things, and perhaps what they also *call* straight things, as bent or curved. Here again, a causal theory of visual perception provides a general explanation of the similarities and differences between the shape-experiences of different people under the same conditions or of the same people under different conditions. The stick appears to be bent when partly immersed in water because the light rays reflected from the immersed part are refracted, or bent, at the surface of the water. It appears to be curved when we put on special spectacles because the lenses distort the light rays. Are we then to take it that it makes no sense to say that the stick *has* a particular shape, or even that it has a shape at all?

It might be thought that this is a hasty conclusion. For it seems to be necessary, in order to explain why we see the stick as bent when it is half-immersed in water, to assume that it really *is* straight. If we draw a diagram to show the refraction of the light rays at the surface of the water, we have to include a line which represents a straight stick. Only so can we explain why it appears to be bent. But does this fact amount to an assumption that the stick *is* straight, in the sense that it *has* just that property which it is perceived to have in normal circumstances? It seems, rather, that what we take for granted when we draw the diagram is not that the stick is straight, in that sense, but that it would be perceived to be straight by a normal observer if it were wholly within the same medium, namely air. Thus, the straight line on the diagram represents the way the stick would be perceived in normal circumstances; and what the diagram then shows is why it is perceived differently in different circumstances. But there is nothing in this account which presupposes that the stick really does have a feature, straightness, which resembles the straightness which it is observed to have when it is perceived wholly within one medium.

In general, what the causal theory of visual perception will tell us is that the stick has some property which is a necessary condition for a normal observer to see it as straight, bent or curved, under specified conditions, or for an abnormal observer to see it in whatever way he does see it under varying conditions. Seen-shape, then, like seen-colour, is an effect; and the theory will allow us to correlate a certain feature of the object with it, but can it be said that this feature is a *shape*? The word 'shape' like the word 'colour' takes its meaning from perceptual experiences, so how can it be applied meaningfully to unperceived factors which contribute to the cause of those experiences?

It is not only colour and shape which present a problem, but the totality of visual perception. If we look at a pencil and cross our eyes, we see two pencils; but there are not two pencils there. We might describe this by saying that when we cross our eyes we see two images of a pencil, or two pencil-appearances. But now, when we uncross our eyes, the two images merge into one; not, surely, into one pencil, for images cannot merge into pencils, but into one image of a pencil. Yet when we uncross our eyes we are experiencing normal vision. So under normal vision, we do not see a pencil directly, or indeed any object, but only an image of it.

There is of course something funny about this argument. For we need the word 'image' to mark just those kinds of odd perceptual experiences which occur when we cross our eyes; indeed it takes its meaning from such contexts. So if we use it to describe all perceptual experiences it is being used in a new, metaphorical, way. It loses its old meaning, which is tied to noticeable perceptual differences, yet no new meaning has been supplied for it. We seem to be trading on emotive associations – images are not quite as good as the real thing

– to make an emotional point with no real content. And if we do insist on using it in this new way to describe all perceptual experiences, by saying that we never see pencils, cats, trees, or whatever, but only images of them, we shall still need to mark those odd experiences which occur when we cross our eyes and we shall have to invent a new word to take the place of the old word 'image'. So it seems that if we call all perceptions images, the only thing we achieve is a change in the language without succeeding in making any real point about the world.

Yet there is a real point to be made, however difficult it may be to describe. It is that double-vision perception and normal perception are *both* experienced effects, and to that extent of a kind. If we take the causal theory of visual perception seriously, then we never see objects directly, either in normal or abnormal circumstances, but only indirectly by way of the effect they have upon us. Light rays strike the object, are reflected to the eye and then pass to the brain; we then experience what we call seeing an object. When we cross our eyes, we introduce an intervening cause, or equivalently, we remove one of the necessary conditions for normal vision and so see double. The effect of the light rays on the eye and the optic nerves is distorted by the unusual position of the eyes in relation to each other. So the theory explains double vision as a distorted effect. For this explanation to carry conviction, however, it has to be accepted that the totality of what we see, under both normal and abnormal conditions, is an *effect* – whether we call it an image, an appearance, or just an effect. When we ordinarily say that we are seeing the pencil, we are experiencing a normal effect; when we cross our eyes and say that we see two pencils, or two images of the pencil, we are experiencing a distorted, or abnormal, effect. In that sense normal visual perceptions and abnormal perceptions *are* of a kind. Yet if that is so, we never see objects directly.

But surely we do experience objects directly in other ways? We can *feel* that the stick is straight whether it is in water, out of water, or partly immersed; and this justifies our saying that it *is* straight, though on some occasions it is seen as bent. Does it? When we run our fingers over the surface of an object it may feel smooth, yet to someone else it may feel rough. Some people have a more sensitive sense of touch than others; indeed the surface may feel both smooth and rough to the same person if he runs different fingers over it. So is the surface smooth or rough? And even gross differences in feelings of touch may be experienced by people under drugs: the stick may feel bent to one such person and straight to another, or straight to one person when he is sober and bent when he is drunk. In what way, then, is the sense of touch different from the sense of sight? We have the same kind of anomalies and, it seems, the same kind of need for a causal explanation. We may say that the object has some property which is capable of triggering electrochemical processes in our nervous system so that we experience the effect which we call a feeling of smoothness or a feeling of straightness, and we can then explain why different people under the same conditions or the same person under different conditions have different experiences. But then, feeling-straight and looking-straight are alike in being effects and neither tells us anything directly about those features of the object which stand as part of the cause.

That a stick feels straight is not evidence that it is *straight*, or even, that it has a shape at all. For again, 'straight' and 'shape' are words which take their sense from what we *experience*, so what sense can they have when used to describe features of causal factors which are not themselves experienced? When we feel that an object is straight, we do of course go on to say that it is straight. But if we take this remark to be describing an actual feature of the object, we should not make the mistake of thinking that the feature which is being referred to resembles the perceived feature. For there is no evidence of that. We do not perceive both the cause and the effect and make a comparison. The most we can say is that the object has some feature which can be correlated with the feelings of straightness which normal observers have in normal conditions, with other feelings which other observers have in other conditions, and so on. There is no difference in kind between the sense experiences of sight and touch; both are effects of unperceived causes and neither gives us direct evidence of what the object is like.

It is not only sight and touch of which this is true. All the sense experiences we have are the effects of unperceived causes.

When we say that an object is hot, or that it is cold, we are not describing some perceived feature which it has. For it might be perceived by one person to be hot and by another to be cold. In such a case, is the object hot or is it cold? Indeed the same person might have experiences of both heat and cold from the same thing at the same time. If we cover one hand with ice and hold the other in front of a fire, then plunge both into the same bowl of tap water, the water will feel hot to one hand and cold to the other. But the water is not both hot and cold.

Such experiences can be explained by a causal theory of perception, but only if it is accepted that feelings of heat and cold are effects caused by features of the object which are not themselves perceived. There is a property of the water which can be correlated with what we feel, or with what we see when we put a thermometer in the water. The molecules are moving about rapidly in water which shows a high reading on the thermometer, or which feels hot in normal circumstances; and they are moving less rapidly in water which shows a lower reading, or which normally feels cool. The effect which this molecular movement has on us then depends on the state of our receptors, so if one hand has been covered by ice and the other held before a fire, the effect will be different on the receptors of the two hands. In this way we can explain the anomaly that the water appears to be both hot and cold. But the state the object is in, the rapidity or otherwise of the molecular movement, is not itself the felt heat or cold. The molecular movement is that feature of the object which causes us to have a feeling of heat or a feeling of cold, and which causes the mercury in the thermometer to expand or contract. We might perhaps feel inclined to say that the object *has* a temperature and that its temperature just is the molecular movement. Or we might say that the object *is* hot (or cold) and then identify *its* heat with the molecular movement. But if so, the temperature of an object, or the heat it has, is not the perceived heat. For in so identifying it, we characterise it as one of the factors which cause our perception of heat.

When we feel the heat from a fire, we believe that the heat is in the fire, or that the fire is hot, or that we feel the heat *of* the fire – *its* heat. But if we put a hand in the fire and feel pain, we do not believe that the pain is in the fire, or that the fire has pain, or that we feel the pain of the fire – its pain. We recognise the pain for what it is, a felt experience which is caused by the fire. In the same way, felt heat is an experience which is caused by the fire. There is no more reason to think that the heat of the fire resembles the felt heat than there is to think that the 'pain' of the fire – whatever it is that is causing us to feel pain – resembles the felt pain.

It might be replied to this that we have put the emphasis in the wrong place. For what is important is that we do recognise a difference between felt heat and felt pain. If our experiences of heat and pain are of the same kind, why is it that we believe the fire to be hot but do not believe that the pain is in the fire? There must be some perceptual basis for this distinction, and perhaps a basis which justifies a general distinction between direct perception, the perception of objects as they really are, and indirect perception, the perception of effects which they have on us. What seems to happen as we put a hand before the fire and move it closer, is that the heat we feel grows in intensity until *it*, the heat, causes us to feel pain. May we not say that the rapid molecular movement in the coal causes the *coal* to be hot and that *the heat of the coal* then causes us to feel heat or, if we are too close, to feel pain? Perhaps; but what is there in this to justify the belief that the felt heat resembles the heat of the coal?

When we smell the characteristic odour of cheese, it is because particles in the vapour rising from it strike the nose and affect the nervous system. In what sense, then, can it be said that the odour is in the cheese or that the cheese has an odour? It has some feature which causes most of us to smell a characteristic odour, but there is nothing to tell us that this feature is an odour; and similarly with its taste.

When we hear the noise of a car, it is because sound waves, caused by the vibrating engine, strike the ear drum and set up vibrations there which are converted to electro-chemical processes. But here our language is less misleading. We do not say that the car has a noise but that it makes a noise. That is exactly what it does: it sets up vibrations which cause us to hear a noise. We do of course say that the car *is* noisy, even if there is no-one there to hear it or if the engine is running in the presence of a deaf man. We might indeed say that the car is noisy, or that it is a noisy car, when the engine is not running. But such remarks are simply shorthand ways of saying that the vibrating engine is generating sound waves in the surrounding air, or that the engine would so generate them if it were running, and that these sound waves would cause a normal observer to hear a noise in normal circumstances. We do not take such remarks to imply that the car *has* a noise. By contrast, if we say that the car is coloured, or that it is a coloured car, we do seem to accept the implication that it *has* a colour. But if objects appeared to be coloured only occasionally, as they appear to make noises only occasionally, we might never have made the mistake of thinking that objects have colours. Or if objects always made noises, as waterfalls do, we might have made the mistake of thinking that they have noises.

We seem to be pushed into a general causal theory of all perception in order to explain the similarities and differences between the experiences of different people, or of the same people in different circumstances. But the explanation entails a sacrifice. If we accept it, we also have to accept that we never perceive objects directly and so never have direct evidence of what they are really like. For the whole thrust of a causal theory of perception is to explain what causes our *perceptions*, from which it follows that the cause is not only not perceived but is in principle unperceivable. If we could perceive it, it would be a perceptual effect itself in need of explanation, not a cause which stands as part of the explanation.

But we might be jumping to conclusions here. Suppose it is true, as it seems to be, that when we have a particular perception – we hear a sound, say – we do not, in the having of that perception itself, perceive what is causing it. Does it then follow that objects, or more particularly those features of objects which stand as causal factors of our perceptions, are in principle unperceivable? We can, after all, perceive directly the vibration of a car engine (which causes us to hear a noise): we can see it. But that is not a way out. For what we see, the shaking engine, is itself an effect caused by light rays which are reflected from the engine and trigger off electrochemical processes in our bodies. We can correlate the two perceptions – the heard sound and the seen movement – but it is not the *seen* movement, the visual experience we have, which causes the heard sound. Both are effects which certain physical events are having on us. But we do not, and cannot, perceive those physical events directly.

Still, it might be said, there is nothing in the causal account of perception which forces us to the conclusion that objects, or those features of them which stand as part of the cause of our perceptions, are in principle unperceivable. To get to that conclusion from the fact that we do not perceive objects directly, we need the additional assumption that if we do not perceive something directly, we do not perceive it – and indeed cannot in principle perceive it. But suppose we say that when we see a colour we *are thereby* perceiving the molecular surface structure of the object, though we are not perceiving it *as* a molecular structure; we are perceiving *it* as colour. Or again, suppose we say that we *do* perceive the molecular movement in a bowl of water which feels hot, but we do not perceive it *as* molecular movement; instead we perceive *it* as heat.

Does this help? This way of describing the situation would not of course allow us to say that we perceive objects directly. For what is meant by saying that we do not perceive objects directly is just that we do not perceive them as they are. But it would at least allow us to say that we do perceive *objects* and, in a curious way, that we perceive some of those factors which cause our perceptions. For in *having* the perception, we *are perceiving* part of the cause, though we are not perceiving it *as* a cause, or as it is. If this is so, however, are we similarly entitled to say that we perceive other factors in the cause? After all, the movement of the molecules in the water is simply one of the factors in the total causal process which results in our perception of heat. Other factors are the electrochemical processes in the nervous system of the perceiver. It is the interaction of certain properties of the object with our bodies which causes us to have a feeling of heat. So is it true that when we feel heat, we are perceiving the molecular movement of the water (though not as molecular movement) and that we are *also* perceiving the appropriate electrochemical processes in our body, though not as electrochemical processes? Consider an analogy. When we perceive the movement of the iron filings towards a magnet, are we thereby perceiving a magnetic force, though not as a magnetic force? Is it true in general that when we perceive an effect we thereby perceive the cause, though not as a cause? If it were so, the problem of causation would look very different.

It is not clear what this way of describing perceptual experiences amounts to; it is not even clear that it is an intelligible way of describing them. But even if it makes sense, it does not seem to get us out of our earlier difficulty. For if we ask whether a given *object* is red, warm, smooth and hard, it is no more helpful to be told that we perceive one of its features as red, another as warmth, and so on, than it is to be told that we do not perceive its features but only the effects which they have on us. In neither case are we told what the *object* is like. In each case we have to accept that we do not perceive features of the object directly, as they really are. But that is where the puzzle lies.

It might be objected to all of this that we have got ourselves into an impossible position because we have missed the obvious. By concentrating on the anomalies of perception, we have ignored the fact of sensory corroboration which characterises most of our experiences. And, it might be said, if we take sensory corroboration into account, there seems to be good reason to believe that, in general, we do perceive objects directly.

Consider again the stick which appears to be bent when it is half-immersed in water. When the stick is out of water, our visual experiences and our experiences of touch corroborate each other. The stick looks straight and feels straight. When it is half-immersed, however, there is a conflict between what we experience by touch and what we see. In the one case the corroboration seems to be good evidence that the stick *is* as it is seen to be – straight; in the other case the conflict is good evidence that some special factor is at work which accounts for the fact that though it is straight, it is seen as bent. And this conclusion is not simply based on an assumption that touch is somehow more reliable than sight. Instead, it depends on the fact that, in this particular case, there is a constancy in what we feel by touch over a range of conditions together with the fact that we have visual corroboration in some of these conditions. The stick feels straight when it is in the water, as it is pulled out, and when it is fully out – at which point our visual perception confirms what we feel, as it did before the stick was put into the water in the first place. It is this which persuades us that the special factor which is at work must be affecting our visual perception, rather than our sense of touch. So we go on to say that the stick *is* straight and *appears* to be bent when it is half-immersed. But if the facts were different, if it felt straight in water and bent when not in water but looked bent under all conditions, then it would be reasonable to take the sense of touch as being affected by the special conditions and we should have good evidence for saying that the stick is bent though it feels straight when half-immersed.

The facts seem to be similar in the case of double vision. We feel one pencil, whether or not our eyes are crossed. That is why we say that in normal vision we see a *pencil*, not an image of a pencil, but that we have a double *image* of it when our eyes are crossed. In this respect most visual experiences differ from simple colour perception, for there is no independent way of observing a colour – red does not have a distinctive feel, but the shape of something solid does. And because our perception of shape is not just visual, so it seems to be a different kind of feature from colour and one which an object can be truly said to have.

Perhaps it makes no sense to say that an object has a colour but it does seem to make sense to say that it has a shape because the evidence here is different. And this is so generally. When we see a white object from a distance, which we take to be a stone, but on walking closer find that it is a sheep, we might be puzzled. We might say that the kind of evidence we have in both cases is exactly the same: a visual perception. So how can the perception itself be evidence of what is there? If it is now correct to conclude from 'I see (what I take to be) a sheep' to 'There is a sheep', why is it incorrect to conclude from 'I see (what I take to be) a stone' to 'There is a stone'? We use the second visual perception to reject the conclusion from the first: we say that we made an erroneous judgment or that our eyes deceived us. But what justifies this if the kind of evidence is exactly the same in both cases – why not use the first perception to reject the conclusion from the second? The answer is that nothing justifies it if the evidence is the same in both cases. But it never is. When we get nearer to the object we see much more detail, and we can relate this detail to other similar experiences we have had of sheep in the past: we draw on the general coherence of our sensory experience. Not only this, but the nearer we get to the object, the more corroborative information we get from our other senses. We can hear the bleating and smell the animal; eventually we can reach out and feel the wool. It is the constancy and coherence of our experiences over a range of conditions, and especially the coherence of the evidence we have from different senses, which seem to justify our belief that in some respects at least we perceive objects directly – in the sense that we perceive features which they actually have.

But do they justify the belief or merely explain why we happen to have it? It is true that these factors, especially sensory corroboration, are at work all the time in forming the judgments we make about the world. The uniformity of our sense experiences on different occasions and by way of different senses provides us with criteria for distinguishing what we call objects from images and illusions. But that is a distinction which is made *within* the perceptual world. Here, however, the problem is different: we want to know whether sensory corroboration, and the general coherence of our perceptual experiences, is evidence that we normally perceive objects directly. For that to be so, the evidence we have by way of sensory corroboration must be different in kind from that which we have from a single visual experience. But though the evidence is different, and there is more of it, and it is certainly understandable why the general coherence of our sensory experience should be psychologically persuasive in leading us to believe that we perceive features of objects which they actually have, how could it be different in kind? How could it provide us with grounds for saying that, when the senses corroborate each other, the object is as it is perceived to be? If every perceptual experience is an effect, what difference does it make that more than one sense is involved and that there is corroboration? What we experience are corroborating effects; but if no one perceptual effect is by itself sufficient to justify the belief that one of the causal factors resembles it, several together are not.

And yet, if this is so, we seem to be in the position of saying that our senses always deceive us. We come to believe by way of sense experience that objects have those kinds of features we perceive, yet it now seems we have no grounds for this belief. Our senses always mislead us as to the true nature of objects. And there is something odd about this. When we see the stone which turns out to be a sheep, we say that our eyes deceived us. But in saying this we imply that our other senses, including our eyes, did not deceive us on a later occasion. The word 'deceive', when used to describe the senses, takes its meaning from situations in which one perceptual experience is classified as deceptive in terms of others which are presumed to be non-deceptive, so it only has meaning if there are situations in which we can rely on our senses. Sense deception is therefore a part of perceptual experience which is resolved by other perceptual experiences. It seems to mean nothing to say, or at any rate there could never be evidence for saying, that our senses are deceiving or misleading us all the time, or that we can never rely on our senses. For there is no way in which the deception or the unreliability could be detected. We are making no new distinction and at the same time losing the old one. It is like calling everything an image. And just as the use of the word 'image' to describe all perceptual experiences is at best metaphorical, so too, the use of the word 'deceptive' to describe them all is metaphorical. But just as there is a real point to be made with the one, so too, in the case of the other; and it is the same kind of point extended now to all perceptual experience, namely that *every* perception is an effect and that there is no evidence whatever that the cause, or any part of the cause, in any way resembles the effect.

If we take the scientific story further, it is not merely that there is no evidence for the belief that objects have features like those we perceive, but that there seems to be evidence against it. If the scientists are right, objects are loose collections of atoms, more space than matter, not solid chunks of material with smooth or rough coloured surfaces. So in saying that our senses always deceive us, we are perhaps doing no more than point to such a possibility in an admittedly metaphorical way – and without wanting to deny that the word 'deceive' takes its meaning from perceptual contexts and is still required to distinguish different kinds of perceptual experiences. Even so, we should not make the mistake of thinking that the scientific account of objects is based on direct evidence of what objects are like. Suppose we could look through a microscope at the surface of a table and see the atoms. We should be having a perceptual experience no different in kind from that which we have when we look at a table without a microscope. What we experience, with or without a microscope, is an effect. So how could this give us information about what the surface of the table is really like? Bigger and better microscopes will not solve this problem. There is no way in which we could perceive any part of the cause of our perceptions however cleverly we devise our instruments. To the extent that a scientific description of objects is perceptual, it is not a description of objects; to the extent that it is a description of objects, it is not perceptual but theoretical. The scientific account of the nature of objects is *based on* perceptual evidence, as our naive beliefs are, but it is a theoretical account designed to explain that evidence, and is certainly not established by direct perception of what objects are really like.

Could we ever know what objects are really like? Of course not; it is self-contradictory to suppose that we could somehow step outside our perceptual experiences to perceive what is causing them. If we could know, we should have to have some non-perceptual evidence. But all our evidence is perceptual. It is not that our senses always deceive us, but that we cannot know whether they do or not. Both the scientific account of objects and our naive beliefs are alike in being theories about the world. When we perceive a piano in a room, we expect to perceive it again in the same way when we walk in next time, and we normally do. The belief that the piano has been there all the time and that it has a certain colour, size, shape and smell, enables us to make this prediction and at the same time explains why the two perceptual experiences are similar. But such a theory does not adequately explain perceptual anomalies; in this respect a causal theory which presupposes the independent existence of objects but which does not entail a commitment to the identification of the piano's features with its perceived features, is much better. It takes into account more evidence and it has greater explanatory and predictive power. For each, however, the evidence is of the same kind – it is perceptual; for neither is the evidence conclusive. So although the scientist's way of describing the world is a theory about it, so too is our ordinary way of talking. We never could have anything but a theory, for we never could have anything other than indirect evidence.

If we cannot know what objects are really like, how do we know that they are there at all? People can be made to 'see' by having their brains electrically stimulated; some people have hallucinations and not only 'see' but 'touch' objects which are not there; when we dream, we might have all the same kinds of perceptual experiences which we have in waking life, but no objects are causing them. May it not be that all our sensory experiences are caused by something other than objects, and perhaps not by anything outside our own bodies? May it not be that there is no cause at all? For if we say that every perceptual experience is an effect, and if the cause is unperceivable, how do we know that there is a cause? Perhaps there are just perceptions – uncaused. For if we can know nothing about the cause, what does it add to our knowledge to say that there is one? What information are we being given when we are told that perceptual experiences are *effects*? But if we go so far, then since my perceptions are mine, private to me, there is nothing but *my* perceptions. Objects, other people, even my own body, I believe to exist because of the perceptions I have of them; but if there are just perceptions, then objects, other people and even my own body are just perceptions which I alone have.

But it is surely not being suggested that because some people have hallucinations and claim to see objects which are not there, or because we all dream from time to time and have experiences which are quite like (and quite unlike) experiences which we have when awake, though no objects are causing them, so all experience might be hallucinatory or dream-like? To take such a view is to use language like putty. The point about hallucinations and dreams, like images, sense deception and illusions, is that they depend on distinctions *within* the perceptual world. This whole way of arguing, or of trying to describe the totality of perception, is fundamentally misleading because it not only has no content, but cannot have a content. Supposing, for the moment, it is possible that there are no objects which contribute to the causal processes of perception and yet our experiences are exactly the same – indeed they have to be, otherwise the argument loses its point. Still this does not put all experiences on a par with hallucinations. For some people would still have unusual experiences which we should want to mark by calling them hallucinations; and the same is true of dreams. There would still be a need, that is to say, to make a distinction between the ordinary perception of 'objects' and hallucinatory perceptions; and there would still be the same differences.

Hallucinatory experiences are characterised by the fact that someone claims to be seeing, touching, smelling, tasting or hearing an object which other observers cannot perceive at all; dreams by the fact that the dreamer has experiences of 'objects' which others who are standing beside him and who are awake do not experience – quite apart from the fact that dream experiences are usually chaotic and lack the coherence of normal life. So the fact that some people have hallucinations, dreams, or induced perceptions caused by tinkering with the brain, cannot in any way be used even as suggestive support for the view that all the perceptual experiences of everyone are hallucinatory.

We might perhaps agree that to describe everything as an image is a suggestive, though metaphorical, way of pointing to the fact that all our perceptual experiences are alike in being effects, but no similar argument from hallucinations and dreams can be used to make the suggestion that they are all alike in being effects of something other than objects. For we need the idea of an object to distinguish hallucinations and dreams from normal experiences, even if the object is nothing like what it seems to be. Both our ordinary beliefs and the causal theory of perception explain dreams, hallucinations and the like as experiences which do not depend on the presence of the perceived object, while normal experiences are those which do. Hallucinations and dreams are therefore an integral part of each theory, not experiences which stand in opposition to them and somehow represent a threat to their credibility.

Of course the causal theory provides a much better explanation than our ordinary beliefs, especially in the case of induced perceptions. In fact, because the causal theory only characterises objects as one of the causal factors of our experiences and takes into account features of the nervous system, we can predict that someone will 'see' if his brain is stimulated in a certain way. But this kind of prediction is justified in terms of the general theory which explains ordinary perception in terms of a causal interaction between the nervous system and independently existing objects. If the presumed independent existence of objects were dropped out of the theory, it would still be necessary to posit some other factor in the causal explanation of our ordinary experiences which is absent in the case of dreams, hallucinations and induced perceptions, in order to explain the perceived differences. Merely to drop out the idea of an independent cause of our ordinary perceptions would give us an emasculated theory for which there is no evidence and which has neither explanatory nor predictive power.

Still, it might be said, a theory of perception which does not pre-suppose the existence of objects, though perhaps a bad theory in terms of its explanatory and predictive power, is nevertheless a possible theory. Our naive beliefs represent a better theory, and a causal theory is best of all, but to say this is to say that all three are alike in being theories. No doubt it is sensible to choose the most useful, but what we want to know is which is correct. How could usefulness be a guide to this? Even in terms of the causal theory we have to accept that in the case of some of our ordinary perceptions of objects, there may be no object there. If the light from a star takes ten thousand years to reach us and if the star exploded yesterday, we shall still 'see' the star, and so will our descendants for the next ten thousand years, though it no longer exists. So it is possible that when we say we see an object, even though we are not dreaming or having an hallucination, the object does not exist; and if it is possible in the case of some ordinary perceptions, why not all?

But this is a bad argument. It certainly makes sense to say in terms of the causal theory that we are seeing a star which no longer exists, but only as a consequence of the fact that there was initially a star there which exploded. If the star had not existed in the first place, we should have to say that the light comes from nothing; and that does not make sense in terms of the causal theory. Not only this, but the theory enables us to predict that in ten thousand years our descendants will see the star explode and thereafter will not see it at all. No such prediction can be made from a theory which denies the independent existence of objects. Such a theory is not, as it were, a simplified form of a causal theory; instead, it is incompatible with it. And because it is, so no conclusions which can be drawn from the causal theory – such as that we are now seeing a star which does not exist – can be used in support of it. Since light from any object always takes some time to reach us, it is possible in terms of the causal theory that every object ceased to exist a moment ago and that there is a split second in which every object we perceive does not exist. But again, in terms of the causal theory, we should soon know it; whereas in terms of that theory which simply drops out the idea of an object, we never should.

That we can never perceive objects directly, and that all our knowledge of what objects are really like is inevitably theoretical, cannot lend credibility to a theory which denies their existence. For these are consequences of a theory which presupposes the existence of objects. It is not simply that a causal theory provides a better explanation of our perceptual experiences, but that it provides a quite different kind of explanation which is inconsistent with a no-object theory. So it cannot in any way provide support for a no-object theory; and if it cannot, what can?

Chapter 4

MIND AND BODY

Do we have minds? There seems to be plenty of evidence that we do. We can feel happy, sad, worried and excited, think wild and wicked thoughts, solve arithmetical problems, understand complicated arguments, make decisions, day-dream, remember, imagine what it would be like to do something we have never done, hope that certain things will happen and others will not, make guesses and fashion secret plans. All such things, we say, go on in the mind, or sometimes, in the head. They are mental experiences or events quite unlike physical events, and even quite unlike those physical events which take place in our own bodies. Feeling nervous is not at all like having a nervous twitch, though the two kinds of events may accompany each other. Having a wild idea is not at all like having a torn ligament. There seem to be two quite different kinds of events: mental and physical.

Why do we want to say that they are different *kinds* of events? An event is a general process applied to, or modified by, a particular object. Moving, printing and painting are general *processes*. Moving a chair, printing a book or a particular page of a book, and painting a picture or a particular bit of it, are *events*: they occur over a definite time interval and in a particular region of space. Similarly, thinking, deciding and imagining are processes; but having a particular thought, making a particular decision and having a particular image, are events which occur over a definite time interval and, in a sense, perhaps, in a particular region of space, since a thought occurs wherever the person is who is having it. But one reason which inclines us to say that mental and physical events are of different kinds is that the 'objects' of mental processes – thoughts, decisions, images and so on – are not themselves physical objects, while the objects of physical processes are. Indeed what seems to make a physical event physical is just that the object is physical, and what seems to make a mental event mental is just that the 'object' is not physical. The movement of a chair is a physical event because, and only because, a chair is a physical object. The movement of an arm is a physical event because, and only because, an arm is physical. But deciding to move an arm or a chair is not a physical event because a decision is not a physical object.

The feelings and thoughts we have, the decisions we make, the day-dreams, hopes and fears, are not discoverable by physical inspection of our bodies. A good doctor will quickly discover my torn ligament or broken bone by feeling the lesion or the swelling; a surgeon who opens me up will be able to see it. But I can sit in my chair and think idly that I ought to be mowing the lawn, and I can decide not to do so; and no-one will ever know unless I tell them. The doctor can prod and the surgeon can slit me open but neither of them will ever be able to feel, see, hear, taste or smell my thoughts or my decisions. If a thought were a physical object, a surgeon could cut it out, look at it, soak it in water and wash the blood from it. It would be a lump of material. And it is because thoughts are not physical objects that we can keep them to ourselves. My thoughts are essentially private to me unless I choose to make them public by producing a physical event such as writing conventional marks on paper. I cannot in the same way keep my torn ligament to myself.

It might be said that this way of looking at things is misleading because it takes the notion of a physical object too narrowly. Of course a thought is not a lump of material – a bit of the brain, say – but it might be a stimulated pattern of brain cells, and in that sense physical. A surgeon could not cut out a pattern and wash it, because a pattern is not a physical thing but it is something which can be detected physically. It is an arrangement of physical things – electrically charged cells; and these can be cut out, washed and stained. But does this make a difference? It may well be true that there are physical brain patterns which accompany my thoughts, and a physiologist who rigs me up to an electroencephalograph will be able to discover that I am thinking by noticing differences in the rhythm of my brain patterns. But he will not in this way be able to discover what I am thinking. He will not, that is to say, be able to discover my thoughts. To suppose that he could would be to suppose that to every distinct thought which it is possible to formulate, there is a unique and detectable brain pattern. And even if this were so and the physiologist or surgeon could always tell me correctly what I am thinking by observing my brain pattern, would he have observed a physical phenomenon which *is* my thought? That to every thought there corresponds a unique physical pattern is no evidence at all that the thought itself *is* a physical pattern.

We can sometimes tell what people are thinking and often find out their beliefs and discover their decisions by observing their behaviour. But this is not to say that we have perceived their thoughts, beliefs and decisions. We perceive certain behaviour patterns which we take to be the effects of certain thoughts and beliefs. But that is to make an inference from the effect to what we take to be the cause. It seems absurd to say that to observe someone's behaviour is to observe his beliefs or his thoughts, even if we can correctly discover them from his behaviour, for that would be to identify the thoughts and beliefs with the behaviour. And it seems to be equally absurd to say that we could observe someone's thoughts by observing his brain patterns even if we could always discover what his thoughts were by observing the patterns.

Of course there are differences in the relations between behaviour patterns and thoughts, on the one hand, and brain patterns and thoughts, on the other. If a man habitually votes for the Communist Party but quite suddenly changes and votes Liberal, we may infer from his behaviour that he has thought about the matter and decided that he was wrong to support the communists. He may even tell us so. But of course he may have decided no such thing. He may be engaged in a deliberate deception. And it is partly because of this possibility of deception that it seems unreasonable to say that observing the behaviour is the same thing as observing the decision. In the case of brain patterns, however, the possibility of deception seems not to be there. If to every decision there corresponds a unique brain pattern, we could not make one decision while deliberately producing the pattern of another, as we can make one decison while producing the behaviour appropriate to another.

Or again, there are cases where our behaviour gives nothing away. What we do may be compatible both with the making of a decision and with not making it, and so cannot be identified with the decision or its absence. If someone decides not to cut the lawn within the next hour, the fact that he does not do so is not evidence that he has so decided. For it may be that he fails to cut the lawn simply because he has not thought about it at all. Sometimes, too, there is no behaviour appropriate to what is going on in the mind. If someone thinks idly about last year's holiday, it is unlikely that his thoughts will be detectable in anything he does. But if every decision and thought has a unique brain pattern associated with it, the presence of a brain pattern would always be indicative of what is going on in a man's mind. So perhaps those factors which make us react against the idea of identifying behaviour patterns with decisions, thoughts, beliefs or whatever, are not paralleled by similar factors in the case of brain patterns.

Yet still it seems absurd to say that a physiologist who is seeing my brain patterns is seeing my thoughts. Suppose there were not these differences between behaviour patterns and brain patterns. Suppose that to every thought, idea and decision there corresponds a unique behaviour pattern and that whenever we observe someone's behaviour we always know correctly what he is thinking. Would it then make sense to say that when we observe the behaviour, we observe the thought? We do of course say that we observe someone's being angry, or even that we observe his anger, but is that to say that we observe his feeling of anger? Surely not; the fact that people can deliberately deceive us by their behaviour, the fact that behaviour is not always indicative of what is going on in the mind, these are only symptoms of what seems to be a fundamental difference in kind between behaviour patterns and thoughts, rather than facts which characterise the difference. The important difference is between what is in principle perceivable and what is not.

I am aware of my thoughts but I do not and cannot perceive them. I do not smell, feel, hear, see or taste them. So how could someone else perceive them? Whoever is having a thought has a direct non-sensory experience of it; and because it is a non-sensory experience, it is essentially a private experience. No-one else can *have* my mental experiences, and no-one, including myself, can perceive them by means of the senses. So any knowledge of my mental experiences which other people have, by observing my behaviour or physical events in my body, must be inferential. Other people can perceive my behaviour patterns and my brain patterns; but just because they are perceiving, so what they perceive is not my thoughts. If it were true that to every distinct thought there corresponded a unique brain pattern, or if it were true that to every distinct thought there corresponded a unique behaviour pattern, it would always be possible to discover what someone is thinking. But this would only be evidence that such patterns accompany such thoughts. It would not be, and could not be, evidence that the thoughts are physical, still less that the thoughts are the patterns. What kind of evidence would establish that?

So what makes us want to say that thoughts, ideas, images, decisions, and so on, are not physical objects, or even patterns of physical objects, is just that they are not perceptible objects to the person who is having them; and from this we take it that they are not perceivable in principle. They are not the kinds of things which can be perceived. And certainly all the rest of our experience is symptomatic of this and fits in with it: we can keep our thoughts to ourselves; we can behave in ways which deceive others about what we are thinking; and we cannot experience anyone else's thoughts. But if a thought is not a perceptible object, or pattern of perceptible objects, then having a thought is not a physical event and thinking is not a physical process even if they are invariably accompanied by physical events and processes in the brain or elsewhere in the nervous system. Having a thought, making a decision and conjuring up an image or a memory are mental events; events which take place in the mind, not the body.

It is not simply thinking, deciding, wishing, hoping, fearing and imagining which go on in the mind. These, certainly, we regard as characteristically mental. But in a sense, any experience we have which involves consciousness or awareness is mental, for being aware of something is a mental event even if it has a physical cause. If I stub my toe and it hurts, I may say that I have a pain in the toe; but I cannot mean this in the sense in which I might say that I have a blood clot in the toe. I may say that the whole toe is painful, but it makes no sense to say that the pain has a volume of one cubic inch as it does to say that the toe has, or that the blood clot has. The doctor can perceive my blood clot, but he cannot perceive my pain. The injury to my toe is the source of the pain, but the pain is not physically in my toe. The particular pain which I am now feeling is something that I and only I am aware of; and it is something which I and only I can be aware of. Someone else may experience the same kind of pain if he stubs his toe, but that is his pain, not mine. When I banged my toe, a causal process began which set up electro-chemical processes in *my* nervous system, and as a result I, and I alone, experienced the effect which is the pain I feel.

So it is with my itches, tickles and tingles. Such experiences are not different in kind from feelings of joy, apprehensiveness or depression, nor are they different in kind from thinking, wishing and imagining. They may seem to be different because in the case of a pain, itch or tingle there may be an obvious physical cause in my body, whereas when I think or feel happy, I do not find a lump on my arm. But in either case, what I am aware of – the sensation of pain or the feeling of joy – is mental, not physical, in spite of the fact that one has a physical cause and the other does not, or at least appears not to have.

If my itches and feelings of pain are mental events, so too are my feelings of heat and cold; for these, too, though they have physical causes, can only be experienced by me. Two people may both touch the same hot poker and both may have the same kind of feeling: if it is very hot they may both feel pain; if it is less hot, they may each have a sensation of heat. But neither has the other's feeling or sensation and no third observer can perceive the feelings they have, though he can perceive their behaviour and infer on the basis of his own experiences what kinds of feelings they are having. So, too, with tastes, sounds, smells and sights. All the perceptual experiences we have are mental effects caused by the interaction of physical objects and our bodies. Two people may look at the same object and both may see the same thing, but neither has the other's visual experience. A visual experience of, say, a chair, is not a physical object, though a chair is; and having a visual experience is not a physical event, though it may have a physical cause.

When we have a thought, our knowledge of it is direct; there is no intermediate sensory process which stands between the thought and our experience of it. We experience it directly. By contrast, our knowledge of objects is indirect because we only experience the effect which they have on us. There is a causal process from the object through the nervous system to the mental experience which is the effect. But, like our knowledge of thoughts, our knowledge of the sensory experiences themselves is direct. We are directly aware of our visual experiences but not of their causes: we do not *see* our visual experiences, we *have* them. To see an object just is to have a visual experience. In a sense, then, we seem to have immediate knowledge of mental events but only inferential knowledge of physical events. The mind, we might say, is more easily known than the body.

Not only this, but the knowledge we have of our mental experiences is essentially ours, inaccessible, except inferentially, to anyone else. The knowledge we have of someone else's mind is like the knowledge we have of bodies – indirect; but the knowledge we have of our own minds seems to be quite different. And it seems to be indubitable knowledge. If we think about a friend, we cannot doubt that we are having the thoughts. We may reasonably doubt whether the white patch on the distant hill is a stone or a sheep, but could we possibly doubt that we are having a visual experience of a white patch? Even if there is neither a stone nor a sheep there and the experience is caused by blurred vision after walking out of a dark room into sunlight, we cannot doubt that we are having a visual experience; we can only doubt the inference we make from it – that it is caused by a sheep or a stone. We may be wrong about what we believe we *see*, but we cannot be wrong about the fact that we are having a particular kind of visual experience.

So not only does there seem to be evidence that we have minds, but it looks as if, in some sense or other, all our conscious experiences are mental. It seems, too, that our knowledge of our own minds is immediate while our knowledge of physical objects, including our own bodies, is not, and that our knowledge of our own minds is essentially private to us and is indubitable.

We seem, then, to know a good deal about the mind, but what sort of thing is it? In one sense, of course, this is a silly question because it is not a thing at all. We sometimes speak of the mind as if it were a kind of box. We say that thoughts, fears, feelings of jealousy and so on, are 'in the mind', but this kind of talk can only be a circumlocution for saying that such experiences are mental.

Just as a thought is not a physical thing, neither is the mind in which it occurs. So, too, when we say that thoughts are 'in the head', we are speaking metaphorically. Neither the mind nor mental processes occur in the head or anywhere else in the body; for being non-physical, they cannot occur anywhere in physical space. If a thought could be located in a physical position, it would have physical properties; it would be a thing of some sort or perhaps an arrange-ment of things. There is of course a sense in which thoughts seem to be locatable in space. For although it is impossible to pinpoint a particular place in my body where a particular thought is, if I go on a trip my thoughts go with me. They take, as it were, an indeter-minate physical location within the space which I occupy. But the reason for this is not that they have a physical location, though an indeterminate one, but simply that they depend for their existence on my existence, and I exist in space. Because I could not exist unless I were in some particular place, no thoughts which I have could exist if I were not in that particular place. But this is not to say that *they* are in that place, it is only to say that I have them: they are mine and no other's.

Yet we seem able to pinpoint them even more precisely. If my brain is taken away, so are my thoughts; for I cannot think without a brain. Even so, though the existence of thoughts depends on the existence of a brain, this is still not to say that they are in the brain. How could a non-physical object be in, literally *in*, a physical thing? It is as if one were to speak into a bottle, close it tightly, and then say that the words are in the bottle. If, when I am having a thought, it is in my brain, where is it when I am not having it? Does it pop in and out of the brain as it pops in and out of my mind? What seems to be true is that there is some connexion, or relation, between what goes on in my brain and what goes on in my mind; but to accept that is very different from accepting that the thoughts in my mind are also in my brain, or more generally in some part of my nervous system. But if what goes on in the brain are physical events and if what goes on in the mind are mental events, what kind of connexion is there between them?

We generally take it that there is a causal connexion. We believe that physical events cause mental events and that mental events cause physical events. If I decide to cut the lawn now, a number of physical events follow. I get up out of the chair, my legs move, I get the lawnmower out, and so on. If we look for the physical beginnings of this causal process, we shall no doubt find it in the brain. Certain brain cells are activated and the resultant electrochemical activity stimulates the appropriate motor nerves which cause the right muscles to expand or contract so that my legs stiffen and I rise from a sitting position. But what stimulates the brain cells in the first place? My decision: and that is not a physical event. If this is so, however, then mental events cause physical events. Similarly, if we trace the causal process by which we come to see, or have some other sensory experience, we shall find the beginnings in some physical causal process between an object and a sense organ – such as light waves striking an object and being reflected into the eye – which excites the sensory nerves and eventually stimulates certain brain cells. This is a physical process which ends with a physical event – the stimulation of the brain cells. But then we have a sensory experience – we see, hear or smell; and that experience is not a physical event. If, however, it is the end of the causal chain then it is caused by the immediately preceding step in the chain, and that was a physical event.

Physical events can cause other physical events: pressing on one end of a lever makes the opposite end move. Mental events can cause other mental events: feeling frustrated can lead to feeling angry. These seem in their own way understandable. They are paired events of a kind. Yet it seems, too, that there must also be causal connexions between events of different kinds, and how can this be? How can something physical bring about something non-physical, or something mental bring about something which is non-mental? For this to be so, it looks as if the connexion between them can be neither mental nor physical, or perhaps, that it has to be both. It is like having a bridge between heaven and earth, one end of which is material stuff and the other end spiritual: how can they meet in the middle?

But perhaps we can avoid this problem by describing the causal process entirely in physical terms. Suppose someone sees a road accident, decides that he does not want to get involved as a witness, and so turns his back and walks away. Up to the moment when he has the visual experience of seeing the accident, the physiologist can give us a detailed story of physical causal relationships culminating in the stimulation of certain brain cells. From the moment he makes the decision to turn away, there will be another complex story of physical causal relationships beginning with the stimulation of certain brain cells. Between the end of the physical sensory process and the beginning of the physical motor process, it looks as if there is a gap which is filled by some quite different kind of activity, a mental process, which the physiologist cannot describe at all in physical terms. So there is a temptation to ask 'What happens in the gap?' and to answer metaphorically by thinking of the mind as a kind of signalman in control of a railway junction, receiving messages about incoming trains and shifting the points so that they depart on the right tracks. But the metaphor is misleading. For physiologically speaking, there is no gap. At every moment of our lives, even when we are asleep, there are physiological processes going on in the brain; and in particular, there is no cessation of brain activity between the sensory impulses which reach the brain when we react to a stimulus and the motor processes which begin when we respond to it. The thinking which takes place 'in the gap' between the end of the sensory causal chain and the beginning of the motor chain is accompanied by brain processes so that, from the physiological point of view, there is a continuous physical causal chain which begins with the stimulus and ends with the response. So there is a complete physiological story which can be given, or which we might reasonably expect could be given when physiology is in a more advanced state than it presently is. Why is this not enough?

Well, for one thing, it leaves out the decision. What takes the place of the decision in the physiological story is the brain pattern which accompanies it, and that, it seems, is something different. If the physiological story is a *complete* causal account of what happens, either the brain pattern has to be identified with the decision or we have to accept that what goes on in the mind is irrelevant to the behaviour. Yet it seems to be absurd to identify the brain pattern with the decision, and it seems to be false that the decision is irrelevant to the behaviour. If the decision is irrelevant to the behaviour, why is it that the thinking which takes place is appropriate to the kind of response which is made? When we decide to do a certain thing – walk away from the accident – that is exactly what happens. Why this particular response rather than some other? It is here that we want to say that the thinking determines the particular response which is made by determining the appropriate brain-cell stimulation. It might be replied to this that it is the physiological brain-cell activity accompanying the decision which determines the stimulation of the appropriate motor cells, not the decision itself; but again, if this is so, it must be the right kind of activity if it is to determine the right kind of response. So it cannot be an accidental accompaniment of the decision, it has to be the right kind of accompaniment. But how can that be if the decision itself does not determine the brain pattern which accompanies it?

At some point we seem to be forced into saying that mental events cause physical events in order to explain the appropriateness of our behaviour in terms of our decisions, intentions and expectations If there were not some *connexion* between the mental activity and the physical processes, how could we ever do what we decide to do? If mental activity is put on one side as a kind of incidental, though apparently related, accompaniment of what goes on in the body, we either have to accept that all our responses are automatic – in the sense that whenever a given pattern of sensory cells is stimulated, a given pattern of motor cells will be – or else that there is some *physical* selective mechanism which determines the right kind of response.

But the automatic story clearly will not do. Some responses, like the immediate withdrawal of the hand from a hot object are automatic and in some sense appropriate. Like the knee jerk, they are reflex actions, but unlike the knee jerk the response is appropriate to the stimulus. It is 'sensible' to move the hand away from a hot object. To say that a response is appropriate to a stimulus, however, is very different from saying that it is appropriate to a decision. Indeed many of the responses we make are inappropriate to the stimulus just because they are appropriate to the decision, for we often make silly decisions. In any case, when we withdraw the hand from a hot stove, no decision has been made; and it is just for this reason that we recognise the automatic nature of the behaviour. Deciding to react to a stimulus in a certain way is the very opposite of reacting to it automatically. But even if we were to drop out the idea of behaviour which is appropriate to a decision and describe what goes on entirely in terms of behaviour which is appropriate to the stimulus, still the automatic account will not do. For behaviour which is appropriate to a stimulus on one occasion may not be appropriate to it on another; and even if it were always sensible to do the same thing in response to the same stimulus, the fact is that we do not always react in the same kind of way in the same kinds of situations. So there must be at least a set of responses from which one is selected. Yet how can the *right* selection be made if the mechanism is entirely physical? If the selection is arbitrary, it seems surprising that so much of our behaviour is appropriate to the stimulus, let alone the decision; and if it is not, we simply have a more complex automatic system.

If an explanation of our behaviour is to be given *entirely* in physiological terms, and if it is not to leave out what seems to be an obvious fact of life – that the way we behave by-and-large matches, or fits in with, our thoughts, decisions, expectations and desires, then we have to accept that these mental phenomena just are the very same thing as certain physical phenomena such as brain patterns, and hence, in the end, that there is no distinction between mind and body. The alternative, which leaves out mental phenomena, processes and events entirely, simply makes nonsense of practically every experience we have. In terms of it, thinking, deciding, wishing, expecting, anticipating, and feeling frightened or dismayed, are irrelevant to our behaviour. They have to be classified as mere accompaniments of our bodily chemistry, playing no part in what we do. It would be as if we were robots whose appropriate responses to stimuli are accompanied by flashing lights which are irrelevant to the physical causal processes going on inside the machine – and not merely irrelevant in the sense that the flashing of the lights does not cause any part of the behaviour, but also in the sense that the flashing is not caused by anything which goes on in the machine. For if we were to allow a one-way connexion, we should be in the position of saying that physical events cause mental events, though not conversely. But if the *whole* story is to be told entirely in physiological terms, there is no place in it for saying that our thinking causes or is caused by what goes on in our bodies – unless, that is, thinking is itself a physiological process.

It might be thought that we can get out of this by saying that mental phenomena and the physiological phenomena associated with them are simply two aspects of the same thing. It is not that there is both a thought and a brain pattern, but just one thing which can be described in two different ways. An electrical discharge between two clouds can be seen as lightning and heard as thunder, but there are not two different things there – lightning and thunder; still less does the occurrence of lightning cause the occurrence of thunder, or *vice versa*. There is just one physical phenomenon, the electrical discharge, though it becomes apparent in two different ways. But this is a bad analogy. It makes sense to say that lightning and thunder are two aspects of the same phenonenon only because we have a third, neutral, way of describing the phenonenon: we can talk about the electrical discharge. There is, however, no neutral way of describing whatever is supposed to 'stand behind' both a thought and a brain pattern. Not only this, but the occurrence of lightning and thunder are both *caused by* the occurrence of the discharge, and the causal explanation can be given entirely in physical terms. So if we are to press the anology, we need a neutral event which is causally related to both having a brain pattern and having a thought, and which is such that the event and the causal connexions can be described entirely in physical terms. We might perhaps feel inclined to say that the neutral event consists of the occurrence of an electrical discharge in the nervous system which causes a brain pattern to 'light up' and a thought to occur. But that leaves us with the problem of explaining how the electrical discharge causes a thought to occur.

Perhaps the analogy is not quite right. Perhaps it is wrong to say that lightning and thunder are two aspects of the same one phenomenon – the discharge. Perhaps the lightning just *is* the discharge, perceived in one way, and the thunder, too, *is* the discharge, perceived in another. If this is so, to speak of the occurrence of lightning and thunder is simply to speak of the same one event – the occurrence of a discharge – in two different ways. There are not three distinct physical phenomena: the discharge, the lightning and the thunder, and certainly not three causally related events. The richness of our language permits us to talk as if there were three things and three events, and it even allows us to speak as if lighting and thunder enter into causal relationships with the discharge and with other things. We say that lightning struck the house or that thunder shattered the window, but we know really that it was the occurrence of the discharge which did these things. So may we not say that electrical discharges in the body just *are* brain patterns *and* thoughts? The occurrence of a discharge does not *cause* either a brain pattern or a thought to occur, and neither the occurrence of patterns nor thoughts enter into causal relationships with each other or with anything else. Having one thought does not cause another to occur; having a stimulated brain pattern does not cause another pattern to 'light up', and the occurrence of a pattern does not cause a thought to occur, or *vice versa*. But electrical discharges do stand in causal relationships to other physical events and only such events. They cause other electrical discharges in the brain or elsewhere in the nervous system, and so cause ligaments to stretch and muscles to expand and contract. Could the story be like this?

If it is, it is nothing new. For if an electrical discharge between clouds *is* lightning, and if it *is* also thunder, then lightning *is* thunder. (Does this mean that we can hear lightning and see thunder?). Correspondingly, if an electrical discharge in the body is a brain pattern and if it is also a thought, then the brain pattern *is* the thought. So we simply have again the position that mental phenomena are identified with physical phenomena. There is no way out of this if the causal story is to be told entirely in physiological terms and mental life is not to be pushed on one side as irrelevant.

We seem, then, to be faced with a choice between the absurd and the inexplicable: the choice between saying that there is no difference in kind between mental events and physical events, or of saying that they are different in kind and yet stand in causal relationships to each other. But if we do not accept one of these accounts, there seems to be no room at all for mental events in a causal explanation of actions.

Why does the idea of a causal connexion between mental and physical events seem so mysterious? Perhaps there only seems to be a problem here because we tend to think of causal relationships as actual physical connexions between physical things. When a golf club strikes a ball, all the components in the event are of the same kind: material stuff. And at the point of impact, there is an actual physical meeting of the club and the ball; they are physically touching. So the description of what takes place can be given entirely in physical terms. Yet there are cases where this is not so even though the objects related are both physical. The causal relationship between the movement of the moon and the movement of the tides cannot be explained in terms of physical contact between the moon and the sea, and the connexion which is taken to relate them, the force of gravity, though it may be construed in physical terms is not a perceivable physical relationship. We can perceive its effects, but not it. If someone strikes us, his fist was propelled by a certain force, but we do not feel the force, only its effect – the blow. Some physical concepts, like force, are essentially mysterious when construed as *physical* properties or relationships. We can indeed in certain cases get rid of such notions by supplanting them with others which seem to have a more direct physical sense. Instead of saying that bodies are attracted by the force of gravity we can say that their movements in relation to each other are due to the curvature of the space around them, and it now seems as if we are talking about a physical property, curvature, of a physical thing, space. But if space is a physical thing, it is a peculiar one. We can see it, perhaps (?), but we cannot weigh it, paint it, or analyse its chemical make-up.

In general, when we talk about the *connexion* in some entirely physical causal relationships, it is not obvious what we are talking about; and it is not obvious that it is always *physical* in the sense in which the related objects are. Perhaps we just take it that the connexion is physical because the objects are; or perhaps it makes no sense to say that it is physical or that it is not. Or perhaps there is just a correlation between two sets of physical events and nothing more. But if that is so, there may be no additional mystery in the relationship between mental and physical events, for we can certainly accept that there is a correlation between thoughts of a certain kind and brain patterns of a certain kind, even though psychologists and physiologists are still a long way from establishing the precise details.

If the causal connexion between two physical events is not entirely without mystery, the relationship between two mental events is certainly not. We do speak as if one mental event causes another. We might say that having a desire for an apple causes us to make the decision to get up and take one from the sideboard. But what exactly is the connexion between two such mental events in purely mental terms? It seems that the content or sense of the desire is in some way connected with the content or sense of the decision. If the desire and the decision are explicitly formulated in words, we can express this connexion of content by way of the meaning or sense-connexion between the two phrases 'wanting an apple' and 'deciding to fetch an apple', but of course such a connexion is not a causal one; and in any case, neither the desire nor the decision need be formulated in words for the one to lead to the other.

Of course, if we could accept the alternative of identifying mental phenomena, processes and events with their physical correlates, we could rid ourselves of two problems at once. We need not seek an explanation of a purely mental causal connexion between two mental events, for those events would be identified with physical events and the causal relationship between them would be physical. Nor need we seek an explanation of the physico-mental causal connexion between a physical event and a mental event; for again, each event is physical and so is the relation between them. The only problem, then, would be to provide an account of purely physical causal connexions, and this seems attractive since we do have some understanding of them. Is this alternative, then, really as bizarre as it has so far seemed? Could it make sense to say that though I do not *perceive* my own thoughts, others can? Well, if there were no reflective surfaces, such as mirrors, I could not in principle *see* my own eyes, though others could. Yet that is hardly an answer. Why is it that if thoughts are brain patterns, we do have a mental life *as well as* a physical one, though computers do not? But perhaps that question begs the main question.

Chapter 5

FREEDOM AND RESPONSIBILITY

Can we ever be held responsible for what we do? We usually think
so and we often justify punishment and reward in these terms. We
send people to prison or even execute them for what they have done,
not merely because we believe that what they have done is wrong,
for we do not always punish people who do something which is
regarded as wrong even when there is a prescribed legal penalty, but
because they have done something wrong and because we believe
they are responsible for their actions. Certainly, a wrong action is
one which we believe people ought not to do, but doing something
which ought not to be done is not of itself enough to justify punishment. If a man is hypnotised, and while he is hypnotised stabs another to death, we do not (or ought not to) hold him responsible.
We say that it was not his fault, that he could not help doing what he
did even though what he did was wrong. We excuse him. We acquit
him of murder, though he has killed.

But what justifies the allocation of responsibility in some cases
yet not in others? We usually make the distinction in terms of a
presumed ability to choose between various courses of action. For we
generally hold people responsibile for their actions only if we are
satisfied that they need not have done what they did. If, that is, we
are satisfied that the circumstances were such that they could have
acted differently. We take it that it is unreasonable to regard someone
as being guilty of a crime unless he had a clear choice between
alternative courses of action and freely decided to do what he did,
or sometimes, if he simply neglected to take an alternative course of
action which he could have taken. For only then can we say that he
was aware of what he did and that he intended to do it or that he
was negligent in doing it. That, anyway, is the ideal, though our
daily judgments and those in courts of law often fall short of it.

Punishment and reward, when considered as a deserved re-
compense for conduct, only make sense if people can be held
responsible for their actions; and responsibility only makes sense if
there is an alternative course of action open and they are free to
choose which course to take. The recognition of diminished responsibility, or of no responsibility in some cases, is an acknowledgment

of the fact that sometimes we are not free to choose a course of action but are instead victims of events outside our control. In some cases, that is, we recognise that a person's actions are caused by something other than a freely made decision and we then excuse what he does. Indeed we might in some such cases say that the person did not in fact perform an *action* because he did not *do* anything of his own volition, rather, something *happened* to him. For 'action' is often taken to mean 'deliberate act', that is an act which involves or presupposes a freely made decision and so entails responsibility. In this sense of 'action' we might say that only actions can reasonably be punished or rewarded, simple behaviour cannot. But however it is described, we do generally recognise a distinction between behaviour which follows from a decision and that which results from some other cause, and the justification for punishing or rewarding the first kind of behaviour, but not the second, is simply that it seems to be up to us what decisions we make, whereas we cannot help doing what we are caused to do. If what someone does is caused by something else, he cannot help doing it; and if he cannot help doing it, he can hardly be held responsible for it.

But in what sense is it up to us what decisions we make? If *every* event is caused, then making a decision is an event which itself has a cause, so how can we help what decisions we make; and if not, how can we ever reasonably be held responsible for anything that we do?

What is it about making a decision which inclines us to say that it is freely made, in the sense that we have a genuine choice between various courses of action? Faced with the choice between an apple and an orange, we feel inclined to say that nothing compels us to choose one rather than the other, or indeed that nothing causes us to choose one rather than the other. But causing and compelling may not be the same. We may feel a desire to taste something bitter, and believing the orange to be bitter and the apple to be sweet, choose the orange. Our choice is then caused by the desire and the belief; but it may not be compelled. Indeed we often feel in such circumstances that in spite of our desires and beliefs we could nevertheless have overcome them and chosen differently if we had wished. And if we had chosen differently, there would equally be a causal explanation of that choice, but still we would not have been compelled to make it. In either case, we feel, whatever we actually do, and whatever the causal explanation of what we do, we could have acted differently.

But the fact is that we did not act differently. We chose the orange. And the decision we made was caused by the desire and the belief we had. So in what sense could we have acted differently? Having just that desire and just that belief caused just that decision to be made; and given those causes, how could the effect have been different? It is true that if the desire and the belief had been different, we might well have chosen differently; but they were not. And given that they were not, were we not compelled to choose in the way we did? No, it might be said, because we can overcome our desires. We can feel a great need to taste something bitter, but nevertheless decide not to yield to our desires. Yet that decision, too, must have a causal explanation. Suppose we believe that too much acid is bad for the stomach and that bitter-tasting things contain a lot of acid. Then, though we may crave the bitter taste, we resist the longing in the interests of our stomachs. So we choose the apple. But that decision is then caused by the desire to look after the stomach and the belief that the orange will harm it. And given these causes, how could the choice be otherwise? To overcome a desire is not to break the compulsion of a causal chain but merely to be compelled by a different chain.

A cause-effect relationship can be suppressed by the introduction of an intervening cause. We can prevent the light from going on when we press the switch by cutting the wires. Is that the sort of thing which happens when we make a choice? Suppose we have a desire and a belief which in normal circumstances would cause us to act in a particular way but that we can choose freely to intervene or not to intervene in this relationship, as we might cut the wires between the switch and the bulb, or not cut them. If we do not intervene then we act in the way which is caused by the desire and the belief; if we do intervene, we act differently. But this is an odd way of looking at it. It makes it look as if *we* are standing outside our own mental life, outside the network of causal relationships between our mental states, but with the ability to pop in and out every now and then to sever causal connexions, as we do stand outside the causal system of power source, switch, wires and bulb yet with the ability to intervene as we please. The analogy makes no real sense. There is no inner agent controlling our mental states, no signalman connecting and disconnecting the points. We, as agents, are not distinct from our beliefs, desires and feelings. And even if the analogy did make sense, it would not explain what a freely made decision is unless we were prepared to say that the choice, to intervene or not to intervene in a causal relationship, is itself uncaused. And how can it be? How can any event be uncaused? An uncaused event would be an arbitrary event having no explanation and no justification. We could only say of it that it happens, nothing more.

If a choice or the making of a decision is uncaused, it just happens. But in that case we can hardly be held responsible for actions which follow from it. Yet if it is caused, we cannot help deciding as we do and again we cannot be held responsible.

There is of course a psychological feeling of freedom. Faced with a choice, we *feel* that we could go either way, that nothing prevents us from going one way or forces us to go another. Even in the case of bizarre choices we still feel this. Given the choice between accepting a million pounds or of being executed, with no strings attached, no threats, promises or coercion of any kind, it may seem inevitable what our choice will be and we may well predict correctly what every person would do when given such a choice. Still, we feel, we *could* choose to be executed *if we wanted to*. But what does this mean? For surely what we want to do – our desire to live – is one of the causal factors in our decision. So all that is being said is that if we had a different desire, the decision would be different. No doubt it would, but that is hardly the point. Since we do have the desire to live, we shall choose the million pounds, nothing could be surer, for the one causes the other.

If the feeling of freedom in such a situation is indicative of some real freedom, it would have to be accepted that though *all* the factors which cause someone to choose the million pounds are present, including the desire to live, nevertheless he chooses to be executed. But how could we ever establish this? We should need to put the same man in exactly the same position twice and see him choose one way on one occasion and the other way the second time. But this is impossible, and not merely in cases where one of the outcomes is as final as an execution. We cannot perform the two experiments with the same man at the same time, and if we perform them at different times some change may have taken place in the interval which affects the decision he makes. There can be no crucial experiment which would settle this question one way or the other.

The feeling of freedom is often illusory. If a man has been brainwashed, he may behave in certain ways which seem to him to be the consequences of freely made decisions, yet we who have brainwashed him know better. He is not responsible for what he does; for despite his feelings, the choices he makes are caused by his previous tutoring. A jury would exonerate him if the facts came to light. How does this differ from what we would regard as a normal situation? Suppose that a man was taught at his mother's knee that oranges are bad for him, though he has long forgotten it, and in consequence always chooses an apple when faced with the choice. He might well feel that he always has a free choice and so could choose to take an orange if he wished. Yet he never does and never would.

If our desires and beliefs are the product of our past experience and training, and if our desires and beliefs cause our decisions, is the feeling of freedom always illusory? Can we ever act in any way other than the way we do act?

One feature of choice situations which might explain the sense of freedom which we have is the fact that, in many cases, the possible choices seem to be equally possible when looked at objectively – from the outside as it were. If we are confronted with a dish containing an apple and an orange and are asked to choose one, there are no external physical restraints which would prevent us from reaching out to take one rather than the other. By contrast, if the apple is contained in a locked compartment of the dish and we are not presented with the key, then we do not have a free choice. Or, as we might say, we are not being presented with a genuine choice because the physical conditions prevent us from acting in one way and force us to 'choose' the orange. So we might feel that when the physical conditions are such that all the choices are equally possible, we are then free to choose.

But there is a fallacy in this way of looking at it. For although the absence of physical restrictions is a necessary conditon for a free choice, or equally, we cannot be said to have a free choice if there are physical restrictions which prevent a course of action, it would be wrong to conclude that when there are no physical restraints, there are no restraints at all. For there may be psychological restraints as equally inhibiting as the locked compartment on the dish. Suppose that we have a strong desire to live and no reason whatever for wanting to commit suicide, and when we are presented with the dish, we are told that the apple contains a large does of arsenic. Are we then free to choose the apple? Physically, yes; but in psychological terms, the choice is not real.

In general, there seems to be little justification for arguing from the equal physical possibility of various choices to their equal psychological possibility, though the appearance of a free choice in a purely physical sense may foster the belief that the choice is free in a much wider sense. The wider sense of freedom, however, may be quite illusory even in the absence of physical restrictions. In any case, the physical conditions of a choice situation are always much more extensive than might at first appear. For we have to take into account the physiology of our nervous systems as well as the external conditions of the situation. If, for example, it is true that a complete causal account of our behaviour can be given in physiological terms, then light reflected from the apple and orange on the plate, and the sound waves caused by the request to choose, together set up sensory impulses in the nervous system which reach the brain and cause motor impulses which in turn cause us to act: the hand moves and grasps the orange. If this is the story, there is no room for choice even in the absence of external physical restraints, and no matter what our psychological feelings. If there is genuine freedom, the decision we make at the end of a sensory causal chain must itself cause a physiological state which *starts* the motor chain; and the decision itself must be uncaused. Yet if the decision is uncaused, we seem forced into saying that it just happens; and if it does, with what justification can we be held responsible for it?

It might be said that the absence of external physical restrictions is all that is necessary to justify a distinction between situations in which we can reasonably be held responsible for our actions and those for which we cannot. If the brakes fail on a car, the physical conditions are such that the driver does not have a genuine choice between stopping or not stopping and so he cannot be held responsible if he runs someone down. So we say that it was not his fault. He could not help doing what he did. We might of course go on to consider whether or not he knew that the brakes were in bad condition, and charge him with negligence if he did, but that is a separate question. By contrast, if the brakes are sound but he still runs someone down, though he had plenty of opportunity to stop, then we might say that he is responsible no matter what he learnt at his mother's knee and no matter what the physiological story about his nervous system.

Yet this seems unjust. If the justification for acknowledging that someone is not responsible for what he does is simply that his actions were caused by forces outside his control, it seems unreasonable to limit these to external forces. And indeed we do not always draw such a sharp line between external and internal compulsions when we allocate responsibility. We are often willing to accept that a man has diminished responsibility or no responsibility because of his mental state or previous background, so where exactly should we draw the line? It has to be shown that cases which we accept as examples of diminished responsibility by virtue of internal compulsions differ materially from those which we call normal, and it is hard to see how to make the distinction. If our mental states and attitudes are caused by our previous experience or by our physiology, and if these in turn cause our decisions, can we ever help doing what we do? Is there a difference in kind, or even of degree, between actions which we regard as involving responsibility and those which we recognise as excusable?

Perhaps we are looking in the wrong place for an explanation of choice behaviour. Perhaps, indeed, it makes no sense to say that our decisions are caused, either by our mental state or by our physiological state. For when we make a decision we seem to be influenced by reasons, and reasons, it might be said, are not causes. Suppose a man decides to buy certain shares. There seems to be a good deal of difference between saying that he was caused to do it and saying that he had a reason for doing it. He might be caused to do it by being coerced by blackmail or threats; in such a case, perhaps, he really has no choice because the coercion is so strong. By contrast, if he is told by his broker that there is to be a take-over bid and in consequence the shares will rise in price, then he has a good reason for buying them, though he is not in any way compelled to do so. In the latter case, we may say, he decided freely even though he had a reason for deciding as he did. For the reason did not in any way cause the decision. He simply weighed up the pros and cons and came to a conclusion.

But is there a real difference here? What the broker told him induced (caused?) the belief that if he bought the shares, he would make money; and he has a desire to make money. Then the belief and the desire together caused the decision. So did he have a real choice? Perhaps the desire to make money is for him just as over-whelming a compulsion as any threat, so that, when coupled with the belief, it was inevitable that he would act in the way he did.

It is not clear that an explanation of decisions in terms of reasons leads to a different kind of account of choice behaviour. Perhaps reasons are not causes; but to accept a reason is to come to have a belief, and beliefs in conjunction with desires can and do operate as causes. There seems in fact to be very little difference between the way a threat operates and the way a reason operates. A threat induces a belief that something nasty will happen, and coupled with the desire to avoid nasty consequences, causes an action. But a reason, too, induces a belief, though not necessarily a belief in a nasty consequence, and so causes an action when associated with a desire. We are more inclined to think of threats as causes simply because threats are usually believed and because we take it for granted that people in general want to avoid undesirable consequences. So we usually pay heed to threats and then tend to think of the threat itself as a cause. But it is no more of a cause, or is as much of a cause, as a reason. Or put another way, a threat is, or can be, a reason for action.

Yet even if we are pushed into accepting a causal account of all behaviour, and in particular, therefore, of choice behaviour, does it make no sense to say, or is it always false to say, that there are some occasions when we have a free choice? We have so far assumed that there is an inevitability about an effect, given its cause. We have taken it for granted that if one event causes another, then whenever the first occurs, the second *must* occur; and if this is so, of course, there is no place for alternative courses of action given an adequate cause, such as a desire and a belief, which will bring about a certain effect.

But it is not obvious where the inevitability lies in a cause-effect relationship. Such inevitability as there is can only be with respect to certain conditions, and since these may be different on different occasions, the effect may be different, even given the same cause. A man may have a strong desire to make money and a strong belief that certain shares will rise, but he can only buy shares if he has enough money; this is a condition which has to be satisfied before the cause can operate. Suppose, then, he does have enough money and he buys the shares, but on a later occasion, faced with a similar situation and having the same desire and belief, he does not do so because he cannot afford it. Does the fact that he chose one way on one occasion and a different way on another, even though the same cause was present, provide us with a reason for saying that on each occasion the choice was free? Hardly; for if an effect is an inevitable consequence of a cause when the conditions are right, then on the first occasion he could not but choose to buy; and on the second occasion, he had to choose not to buy since an intervening cause – the lack of money – prevented him from buying. An appeal to necessary conditions as a way of softening up the inevitability of a cause-effect relationship cannot succeed. For if we take a cause-effect relationship to satisfy the requirement that, if the conditions are right and the cause operates then the effect *must* follow, we have the position that when the conditions are right and the cause operates, the effect is inevitable; but when the conditions are not right that is because an intervening cause is present in conditions which guarantee the inevitability of *its* effect.

The only way of softening up the inevitability of a cause-effect relationship is to show that the same cause, under exactly the same conditions, could on one occasion produce a certain effect and on a different occasion fail to produce it. Thus, we have to deny the general causal principle that the same cause will, under the same conditions, always produce the same effect. This would allow us to accept a causal account of behaviour which at the same time leaves room for the possibility of free choices. Alternatively, we could deny a causal account of behaviour, at least to the extent of accepting that decision-making is uncaused, but that too would be to deny a general principle – that every event has a cause. What we cannot do, it seems, is to accept all the causal principles we normally accept and still insist that there are free choices.

Then perhaps we should simply bite the bullet and agree that, so far as our mental life is concerned, the general principles of causation do not apply. But what would that mean – that some of our behaviour, at least, is in principle inexplicable? Is that why we can be held responsible for it? If so, it seems to be a funny kind of justification for punishment and reward: let us only blame and praise those who do something which cannot be explained. This is not a real alternative. Yet there seems little doubt that the belief we have in free choices does depend on the view that a decision is an uncaused intervention in a causal chain and is such that it can affect the outcome of that chain. And what is so puzzling about this is not so much that a decision can cause or prevent bodily actions, though that is puzzling enough, but rather, that it should not itself be the inevitable consequence of some causal chain.

The attempt to explain decision-making in terms of reasons instead of causes is one way out of this dilemma, but it seems not to stand up. An alternative is to explain decision-making in terms of norms or rules. For we often choose a course of action which we consider to be right in terms of some rule or principle of behaviour even when it goes against our desires. In such cases, it seems, our choice determines a course of action which is the direct opposite of that which would have come about if we had allowed the cause (our base desire) to operate. So we might think that when we act in accordance with a rule, our actions are not caused. But again, may we not say that the belief that a certain course of action is right, together with a general desire to do what is right, causes us to make the decision we do? The other base desire we have, to do the wrong thing, is simply less strong than the desire to do right and is therefore suppressed. Of course this might be a strong argument for indoctrinating people to want to do the right thing, but it is hardly an argument which justifies the belief that our choices are free.

We seem almost to be in the position of saying that we should attempt to cure criminals rather than punish them. For if people can never help doing what they do, what they do is never their fault. But of course we could seek to justify punishment in some other way. We could justify it in terms of revenge, or the protection of society, or even, as part of the cure. For in general people want to avoid punishment and gain reward. So we might use punishment, or the threat of it, to educate them into inhibiting wrong behaviour, and use rewards to reinforce right behaviour, as psychologists use rewards and punishment to teach their rats how to run the maze correctly. And this is not unreasonable if all behaviour is caused, for rewards and punishment, praise and blame, are then simply used as causes to modify behaviour. But if all behaviour is caused, there is no place for responsibility, any more than there is with the rats, for there is no place for the deliberate wrong action, or indeed for any deliberate action.

To deliberate, to weigh the pros and cons, to reach a decision freely and then to act, knowing that it was possible to act differently and being willing to accept responsibility for the decision, all of this presupposes a break somewhere in the causal network. It presupposes the ability to intervene in the course of events and to change it by means of a decision which need not have been made. It presupposes the ability of a god. For the idea of a free agent as a spontaneous intervener in causal chains is an ideal which seems to be unrealisable in space and time. To be in space and time, as we are, is to be subject to causal laws, to be a part of the causal network. To be free of the causal network in some crucial respect, as in the making of decisions, and to be capable of intervening in the natural course of events to bring about a change which would not otherwise have taken place, as we believe ourselves to be, is at least to some extent to be independent of the natural order in space and time, and to that extent to stand 'outside' it. But if the universe is a causal system, if *every* event within it has a cause *within it*, how could we, or any other finite being, intervene from the 'outside'? Yet if we intervene from the inside, in what sense is our action an *intervention*?

Chapter 6

THE EXISTENCE OF GOD

Does God exist? This is not the same question as: Is there *a* god? The answer to that question would be yes if it could be shown that a supernatural being exists, independently of any other properties it might have. But God, the Christian God, though conceived of as a supernatural being, is much more than this. In terms of Christian doctrine, God is unique, all-powerful, all-knowing, infinitely wise, good and intelligent. He is the creator of the universe and he is capable of intervening in wordly situations by bringing about or preventing various events. He is not, however, malicious, envious, jealous, greedy or wicked. And although he has sometimes been endowed metaphorically with physical properties, such as a human form, it is usually held that he does not exist in space and so does not have physical properties. If he existed in space, it would be in principle possible to find him in some particular place – living on Mars, Pluto or some body in an outer galaxy, perhaps – and this, though it might be compatible with some religions, is not part of Christian orthodoxy. It might sometimes be said of course that God lives in heaven; but then, heaven is not thought to be a particular bit of the physical universe, like Pluto. More to the point, perhaps, is the fact that if God created space then some part of his existence at least – that which he had before the creation – was non-spatial. Of course theologians differ on what they think can or cannot be said sensibly about God, but there seems in general to be at least this much common ground, and it seems to add up to saying that God is the perfect mind. To show that God exists, then, is to show that there is a supernatural being which has certain quite specific properties and which fails to have certain other properties.

It has sometimes been thought that God's existence can be demonstrated from his presumed properties. For every property which God is conceived to have is perfect of its kind, indeed God is perfection. Yet a being which fails to exist is less than perfect. Therefore God must exist. But this is scarcely an argument. How could the mere idea of God entail his existence? If we accept that a being which fails to exist is less than perfect, then what can be said is that *if* there is a perfect being, it exists. But that tells us nothing;

for it says only that if there is a perfect being, there is a perfect being. The statement is true, in fact necessarily true; but so, too, is the statement that if it is raining, then it is raining, though it tells us nothing about the weather. Indeed it is just because it tells us nothing about the weather that it is necessarily true: it could not be false whether we have a cloudburst, a hailstorm or a bright sunny day. Similarly, the statement that if there is a perfect being then it exists, could not fail to be false; but that is only because it tells us nothing whatever about the existence of God. If God exists, it is true; and if God does not exist, it remains true.

Arguments of this kind are irrelevant to the question of God's existence, and inevitably fallacious, because they go in the wrong direction. For the problem is not: how can we demonstrate God's existence on the basis of the fact that he has such-and-such presumed properties? It is, rather: how can we demonstrate the existence of a god which has such-and-such properties? We could never argue validly from belief to existence, instead we need to justify belief on the basis of existence. Even in mathematics, which seems to provide the model for this kind of argument, we cannot make such a move. Given the general properties of right-angled triangles we can demonstrate that the square on the hypoteneuse of any such triangle is equal to the sum of the squares on the other two sides, but we cannot establish the existence of right-angled triangles given only their general properties.

It would be equally irrelevant and fallacious to claim that because we might have 'made up' God's properties in some way, this is a reason for saying that he does not exist. It is of course clear that many of the properties which God is supposed to have are projections of human properties. We know what it is like for human beings to have power, to have knowledge, to be wise, good and intelligent. We know what it is like to create things, and we believe ourselves capable of intervening in a causal order and of bringing about or preventing various events. And we can conceive of what it would be like to have more power than we have ever experienced, to have more knowledge, to be wiser, better and more intelligent. So there is a sense in which we could get the idea of God by projecting what we take to be the best of human properties to an ultimate end. We could, that is, conceive of a perfect man, unlimited by birth or death, unhampered by physical properties and conditions, and not restricted by viciousness, malice, greed or envy. We might indeed believe that such a being exists merely because we wish that it were so, for then there would always be someone we could turn to in times of crisis who would do for us what we would do for ourselves if only we were capable of it. But though the idea of God *could* be

THE EXISTENCE OF GOD

the product of wishful thinking, this is not to say that it *is*, still less that God does not exist. For a psychological account of how we might create the idea of God, or even of how we did create it, is irrelevant to the question of whether or not there is such a being. We could create the idea of a fish which has never been experienced and which has, say, twenty fins, but whether or not there is such a fish is a separate question. That is a question which can only be settled in terms of evidence.

Then what is the evidence for or against the existence of God? We know what kind of evidence would settle the question about the fish. It would be conclusive if someone were to present the fish to us on a plate; it would be less than conclusive, but still convincing, if a biologist were to show us that there would be a 'species-gap' in the natural order if such a fish did not exist, or alternatively that it would be incompatible with present biological fact or theory for there to be a fish with twenty fins. But this kind of evidence seems not to be available in the case of God. If God does not exist in space, it is impossible for us to establish his existence by perceiving him; and again, if he does not exist in space, it seems that no scientific theory could be relevant, one way or the other, to the question of his existence. For questions of existence in relation to a scientific theory are always of existence in space and time. Scientists deal, and can only deal, with what is and what happens in the physical universe. So it might be thought that no fact about the world, and no scientific theory based on such facts, could lead us rationally to the conclusion that God does or does not exist.

We might then feel inclined to say that because God, if he exists, does not exist in space, he is not in principle perceivable, and that this of itself is enough to show that he does not exist, or at the very least that there never could be evidence to show that he does. But this is too easy. We believe that there are material objects, physical objects in fact, which, if the scientific causal theory of perception is correct, are not in principle perceivable. For in terms of the theory, our perceptions are the effects of causes, and among the causal factors are objects which cannot themselves be perceived; if they could, they would themselves be perceptual effects standing in need of a causal explanation.

More relevant, however, is the fact that our thoughts are not in space and are not in principle perceivable, though we are aware of them and so have good evidence that they exist. And we certainly do not perceive the thoughts of others and neither are we aware of them, though we believe with good reason that other people have thoughts. That there are thoughts other than our own is an inference we make from the observation of events which are not mental. We

observe someone's actions and infer that he has thoughts because
we take it, on the basis of our own experiences, that the actions are
the effects of thoughts. Indeed we frequently infer to the existence of
unperceived causes, and to causes which are in principle unperceivable, because we take events to be effects rather than happenings
which just occur. All our claims to knowledge of other minds,
including knowledge of their existence, depend on this kind of
inference. But God is conceived to be the perfect mind and it may
not therefore be impossible to arrive at a knowledge of God, and
of his existence, in this way.

Yet though we can perhaps agree that the evidence we have for
the thoughts of others is indirect because they are in principle unperceivable and do not occur in space, nevertheless our beliefs about
them are wordly in the sense that we take them to occur within the
natural universe. For they exist in time if not in space. Whether or
not God can be said to exist in time is, however, a puzzling question.
He is eternal, since he has no beginning or end in time; he is sometimes said to be present all the time; and if he can intervene in
worldly events, then the effects of these interventions are themselves
worldly events which occur in a temporal order and at a particular
time. But whether the causes of these effects, God's decisions to
intervene, say, can be said to take place at a particular time is not
clear. For *they* are not worldly events. Not only this, but since our
sense of time derives from sequences of events which take place
within the universe, and since God is supposed to have created the
universe, there was no time, in our sense, when the creation took
place. We may say, perhaps, that the creation took place before the
temporal order of events within the universe began, but it is not clear
what meaning 'before' and 'began' have here. Again, if God is
eternal, then in some sense of 'before', he existed before the universe
did. So in attempting to describe some of God's properties and
actions we seem pushed into the idea of a super-time, God's time,
in which events occur in some sort of temporal relation to events in
the universe. It might, however, make more sense to say that the act
of creation, and indeed all God's actions, are non-temporal, in our
sense of 'time', as God himself is said to be non-spatial, in our sense
of 'space'. So if we are going to say that it might be possible to infer
the existence of God as a thinking mind on the basis of observations
which we make within the universe, as we infer the existence of
human minds other than our own on the basis of observing non-
mental events, we have to be clear that God's non-temporality may
make an important difference. And we have to be clear, too, about
which events are relevant and why they are relevant.

It might now be thought that the idea that God does or does not exist is absurd. For if God is a non-spatio-temporal being, how could any spatio-temporal or temporal event be relevant to the question of his existence? How could any event which takes place within the universe be relevant to anything outside it? Indeed the notion of something existing 'outside' the universe seems to make no sense.

But there is more to it than this. If the concern were simply to show that a supernatural being exists, but does not have spatio-temporal existence, then no perceptual knowledge and indeed no fact about the spatio-temporal universe could count as relevant evidence either for or against. That is, the question, 'Does a god exist, though not in space or time?' could not be settled one way or the other. The question of *mere* existence, if it cannot be settled in terms of ordinary criteria, such as direct perceptual evidence or evidence drawn from a scientific theory, cannot be settled; at least not by us. It is not, for us, a real question. But the question of whether or not God exists is different. For God is not conceived of as an empty being. He is a particular kind of being with certain properties, and some of these properties, at least, are worldly, or at any rate are supposed to have worldly effects. Though standing outside the spatio-temporal universe, he is supposed to be in some way related to it. He created it and he can change the course of events within it. So if it could be shown, for example, that an event occurred which could not be explained in any way except by presupposing the intervention of God, this would be evidence of his existence. The question of whether or not a particular event is a miracle, therefore, is relevant to the question of God's existence. Or again, if it could be shown that the spatio-temporal universe had no beginning, or if the assumption that it began at a particular moment in time is incompatible with some scientific theory, that would be partial evidence that God does not exist, though it would still be left open whether a god exists which has all the properties of God other than the property of being creator of the universe.

In saying these things, however, are we making the earlier mistake of thinking that God's existence can be demonstrated from the properties which we want, expect or believe him to have? No; what is being said here is different. It is that if God is conceived to have certain properties, and if there is evidence, either direct perceptual evidence or evidence from a scientific theory which is based on perceptual evidence, that certain events cannot be explained except in terms of a being which has those properties, then that is evidence of God's existence, though not of course conclusive evidence. But also, if God is conceived to have certain properties, and if there is evidence that constitutes a denial of the possibility of these properties in any being, then God does not exist, even if a god does. In each case, it is not God's presumed properties alone which are appealed to, but these together with facts about the world. To show that triangles exist or do not exist it is necessary both to know what the properties of a triangle are and to know certain facts about the world – for example that it is or is not possible to construct spatial realisations of straight lines. In a similar way, though the analogy is not exact (we do not, for example, want to show that gods exist in the world), the question of God's existence is a question of the compatibility of God's properties with relevant facts about the world. Is there, then, any evidence of this kind?

It might be said that God's non-existence is incompatible with every fact about the world and with every scientific theory. For every event has a cause, and every scientific theory depends on this fact. But the origin of the universe is an event, so it, too, was caused by some other event. That event, however, the cause of the universe's coming into being, cannot itself be spatio-temporal since spatio-temporal events are those which happen within the universe. There was, therefore, a non-spatio-temporal event which brought about the origin of the universe. It must therefore have been the decision of a non-spatio-temporal being. So there is a non-spatio-temporal being which created the universe.

This is not an argument for the *mere* existence of a non-spatio-temporal being. As we have seen, there can be no worldly evidence relevant to that. It is instead an argument for the existence of a mind-creator, and to that extent an argument relevant to the question of whether or not God exists. But it does not conclusively establish the existence of God, even if it is acceptable, for a decision-making being which created the universe need not be benevolent, all-powerful or wholly good.

Is it a good argument? What is being used as evidence is the fact of a causal order. Because we have, or seem to have, evidence that one event can cause another and that no event occurs without a cause, the mere existence of the universe provides a ground for saying that some event brought it into being – for it must have had a beginning. But it is a puzzling argument. Suppose there is a causal order within the universe. Our evidence for that, such as it is, is based on experience of spatio-temporal events; that is, on events which occur within the universe. We have no evidence whatever of events which do not occur at a place or at a time; and consequently no evidence of causal relationships between such events and those which are in space or time. The idea of a cause, then, is *essentially* worldly. With what sense, then, can we speak of a cause which occurs outside the spatio-temporal universe? It is true that we have, or believe ourselves to have, experience of non-spatial causes. We believe that our decisions cause our actions, and though the actions are spatio-temporal, the decisions are not. So perhaps we have worldly evidence for saying that every event has either a spatio-temporal cause or a temporal cause. In fact we could go further and claim that since some mental events cause others, and since mental events are non-spatial, so we have experience of non-spatial, though temporal, events caused by non-spatial, but temporal, causes. And given such experience, we might say that we can project our ordinary idea of a cause to an ideal and conceive of a non-spatio-temporal cause of an event. But what content does the ideal have if it is divested of *all* its worldly attributes? We are to conceive of the absence of all spatio-temporal events, of nothingness, and presumably, too, there-fore, of the absence of space and time. But then suddenly there is an event: the universe comes into existence. And that cannot simply happen, we say, because nothing can happen without a cause. Yet what we mean is that nothing can happen without at least a temporal cause, and we do not want to mean that unless God can be said to exist in time. But how could he? Does he get older, do his properties change? There are no ordinary criteria which could be applied to show that God is a temporal being.

We cannot of course ask sensibly who or what brought God into existence. To do so would be incompatible with the idea that God is eternal and had no beginning, but that is not the important reason. The real reason is that if the question is sensible it presupposes that we understand what is meant by saying that a non-spatio-temporal event brought into existence a non-spatio-temporal being. For if the universe, and consequently spatio-temporal events, did not exist 'before' God existed, and if an event brought God into being, that event occurred in neither space nor time. That is inconceivable. Yet the only difference between it and the idea that God created the universe is that what is brought into existence is different – in the one case a non-spatio-temporal being, in the other the spatio-temporal universe. The kind of cause, however, is the same: it is an event which cannot occur in space or time.

Suppose we say we know what it is like to create something. Indeed we know what it is like to create something *simply* as the result of making a decision. We can create a melody or a poem in the head. But we do not know what it is like to create something *physical* simply as the result of making a decision. We can paint a picture and so create something which did not previously exist, but it does not come into being as the consequence of an act of will and nothing else. We need materials; bits and pieces which are already in space and time. We create new things out of old, we do not just create, out of nothing. But it might be said that we can conceive of what it would be like simply to think a picture, as we do a poem, and then for it to appear. We can conceive of what it would be like to think of a house and have it appear in the garden. Perhaps we can; but then, the thought occurred in time and the created object appeared in both space and time.

Is what we can conceive or cannot conceive relevant? There is a danger of supposing that what has not been experienced is inconceivable and that what is inconceivable is impossible or even absurd. There is, too, the other danger of supposing that what is conceivable is possible, and that what is possible is. The difficulty about God's properties, and arguments for his existence, is that they not only take us a step beyond experience but a step beyond the possibility of experience. So we are led to consider what can or cannot be conceived on the basis of experience when the real question is whether a step beyond the possibility of experience is a step beyond possibility, into impossibility or absurdity.

It is not clear that conceivability is a test of possibility, or inconceivability a test of either impossibility or absurdity. Of course the conceptions we are able to form depend on our experience, and of course our experience is of spatio-temporal events, but we can to some extent at least 'think away' the spatio-temporality of an event and make some sense of a non-spatio-temporal cause – a bringing into being of something which was not previously there. The creation of the universe, if it occurred, was a unique event, so it is clear that we cannot explain it or even describe it in terms of experiences derived from the occurrence of events within the universe, but we can get some analogical idea of it. And then we might say that since it did occur, it must have been brought about by something – since every event has a cause.

But that belief, that every event has a cause, is in fact the belief that every spatio-temporal event has at least a temporal cause. It cannot have any other sense, yet that is not the sense in which we want to use it. We want to use it in the sense that every spatio-temporal event has a cause, without qualification. And although we might consider that a non-temporal, non-spatial, cause is conceivable, we still may not be making a statement with any real content when we say that every spatio-temporal event has a cause, still less a statement which we have grounds for believing to be true.

Even if it is granted that it makes sense to say that every spatio-temporal event has a cause, without qualification, and even if it is true, it is still not clear that it will carry the weight of the argument. For it is not obvious that the actual coming into being of the universe – the effect of the non-spatio-temporal cause – is itself a spatio-temporal event. The universe is the framework within which spatio-temporal events take place. So how could the origin of the universe itself be a spatio-temporal event? It did not take place *within* the universe, instead it began the possibility of spatio-temporal events. Suppose the universe which was created was simply a speck of dust in space – the rest, the development of galaxies, we can leave to the operation of natural laws. After the creation we can speak of spatio-temporal events. We could say that the speck of dust got bigger and we could use this growth to determine a before and after. We could say, perhaps, that it began to grow the moment it came into being, or a few moments after it came into being. We could, that is, use the creation as a temporal origin and the centre of the speck of dust as a spatial origin to determine a point from which the growth of the speck could be measured. But the actual coming into being of the dust in space was not an event which took place within that framework. So it looks as if the application of the principle 'Every (spatio-temporal) event has a (spatio-temporal or temporal) cause' has to be in the form 'Every non-spatio-temporal event has a non-spatio-temporal cause'; and with what justification do we make that move?

But what is the alternative: that the universe simply came into existence? That it just happened, nothing more? This is not the only alternative. Perhaps it never had a beginning. Yet what would that mean, that it goes back infinitely?

It might be said that infinity makes no sense in terms of material things. We can make sense of it in terms of abstract entities like numbers. We can think of the fractions less than one and recognise that there cannot be a smallest. For we can take a tenth, a hundredth, a thousandth, . . ., a millionth, and since there is nothing which prevents us, at least in theory, from adding further zeros to the denominator, we can see that we can go on creating smaller fractions. We can never reach the smallest fraction; and this is the same as to say that the sequence of fractions less than one, when arranged in order of increasing magnitude, has no beginning. We cannot begin with the smallest and work our way up because there is no smallest. But this is an entirely abstract sense of 'no beginning' arising from the fact that the technique or rule for adding further zeros to the denominator has no temporal restriction on it. It is a non-spatio-temporal rule. In practice, however, we cannot go back infinitely. However we arrange it, however many people we employ to do the job, there are going to be spatio-temporal restrictions on the enterprise and we shall eventually come to an end. It is not clear, then, what the sense of 'could' is in 'We could always go further'; it expresses some sort of ideal or logical possibility, not a physical possibility. In thinking of the existence of the universe, however, we are thinking of spatio-temporal events, and therefore of physical possibilities. We know that the existence of every material thing has a beginning in space and time: nothing has or could physically exist infinitely. And every collection of material things has a beginning as a collection, for the collection does not exist before at least one of its members does. Yet the universe is a collection of material things, so it must have had a beginning. There was no universe when there were no things and no things can exist infinitely.

This is a bad argument. We may grant that if there was a time when there were no things, there would be no universe at that time. However, it does not follow from the fact that no thing can exist infinitely that there was a time when there were no things, and consequently a time when there was no universe. For different things may exist at different times, and even though no one of them exists infinitely, their periods of existence may overlap in such a way that there never is a time at which nothing exists. For a collection to exist infinitely, it is not necessary that any one of its members should. In any case, to say that every material thing has a beginning is to say that it has a beginning in time, that is, a temporal origin *within the universe*. So we cannot mean 'beginning' in the same sense when we say that the universe must have had a beginning.

What, then, could it mean to say that the universe had no beginning? Simply that, for any event we care to select, there is always an earlier event. There is, that is to say, no date in the history of the universe which can be taken as the first. Indeed if there were, we should have to abandon one of our causal principles – the very one which seems to lend support to the argument from creation: that every spatio-temporal event has at least a temporal cause. For if there was a *first* spatio-temporal event, then no such event preceded it, and therefore no temporal event caused it. Consider the created speck of dust which begins to grow. If its beginning to grow is the very first spatio-temporal event, then it had no spatio-temporal or temporal event as cause. If the universe had a beginning, therefore, its creator had both to create it and bring about the first event within it.

This may not seem unreasonable if we are seeking to establish the existence of a god who both created the universe and has the power to intervene in the spatio-temporal causal order. For the initiator, or prime mover, of the causal order might be expected also to have the power of intervention. And indeed it is not unreasonable from this point of view. What is unreasonable, however, is the argument which seeks to establish the existence of a creator on the basis of the belief that every spatio-temporal event has at least a temporal cause. For if there was a creator, that belief cannot be true.

In general, the argument for the existence of a creator which is based simply on the two premisses, that the origin of the universe was an event, and that every event has a cause, seems not to stand up. It fails because it depends on identifying two senses of 'event', a worldly sense and a non-worldly sense. Lying behind the argument, however, are two facts: the fact that there *is* a universe (which, it is then assumed, must have had a beginning); and the fact, or the apparent fact, of a causal order *within* the universe (which, it then has to be assumed, is true of 'events' which do not take place within it). The parenthetical remarks here point to the weaknesses in the argument, but they do not in any way deny the facts which are being relied on. And if these facts are not disputed, they can be used in a different way to support a different argument. For suppose we shift the emphasis and say: it is not the mere existence of the universe which is important. Rather, what is important is the existence of a causally ordered universe. For order reflects, or reveals, a design; and a design presupposes a designer.

The strength of this new argument derives from the same two facts as before: that there is a universe and that there is a causal order within it; but they are exploited differently. The conclusion, too, is different. For even if the argument is sound, it does not establish the existence of a god who created the universe, but rather, of a god who organised it. The difference is that the order might have been imposed on materials which were already there in a state of chaos. Of course, one might seek to take the conclusion further by claiming that the universe was created as a causally ordered system. In that case, the creating god was also, perhaps, the designer. But the argument from design does not by itself support this. Even the two arguments together do not support the stronger conclusion. For there is nothing in either which commits us to the position that the designer has to be the creator, or the creator the designer. The simple argument from design, if it is sound, will at most establish the existence of an intelligent supernatural mind. Is it sound?

What does it mean to say that order reflects, or reveals, a design? Suppose someone who has never seen a watch is presented with one. He observes the regular movement of the hands and he discovers, perhaps accidentally, its usefulness in keeping time. He takes off the back and he observes the intricate relationship between the parts. He sees that the movement of the hands is caused by the movement of a cog, which in turn is caused by the movement of another cog, and so on. And he sees that the whole system derives its power from an energy source, the spring. There seems little doubt that he would recognise this as an ordered system. Everything fits together. It might then seem obvious to him that the watch was designed for the purpose of keeping time. Is the universe like this?

We might consider a human body and notice how each part is useful in contributing to its survival – hands are useful for defence, for food-gathering, and so on. We might consider the arrangement of cells and discover their different specialised functions which contribute to the welfare of the organism as a whole. Or, on a larger scale, we might discover that the body needs oxygen to survive, that there is oxygen in the air which it consumes, and that trees and plants give off oxygen, so replenishing the supply. And we might discover that the whole system derives its power from an energy source, the sun. Everything fits together. It might then seem obvious to us that the cells in our bodies, the organisation of our bodily parts, and the environment in which we live, were designed for the purpose of promoting our survival. The story could of course be elaborated much more, and not only in respect of human needs and conditions.

But what justifies our saying that this is an *ordered* system? What justifies our saying of any system that it is ordered? If anyone throws three stones into the air, they will always fall in such a way that they mark the vertices of a triangle (unless, of course, they fall in a straight line, but that could be regarded as a degenerate case of a triangle). Do they always, then, fall in such a way as to constitute an ordered system? No, it might be said, because the only thing we can conclude from such events is that the stones will fall in some triangular arrangement or other. But to say that, is to say nothing. It would be significant, however, and indicative of an order, if the stones always fell in such a way as to mark the vertices of the very same triangle. This could not happen by chance. Regularities like this are indicative of order, and it is a feature of causal systems that they exhibit such regularities.

Let us grant, then, that a causal system is, in some sense, an ordered system. Still, we may ask, what justifies our saying that the existence of order indicates a design or a purpose? If it is true that we have adapted to our environment, how could it not be true that the environment 'fits in' with our needs? If animals, and indeed species of animals, have died off because they could not survive in the environment as it is, what does it add to say that the environment is suited to those which have survived? What does it add to say that the system was planned so that these things would happen?

The analogy of the watch is misleading. For it is set in a context in which we already know why watches are made. So it comes as no surprise to think that a newcomer to watches would be able to infer from the existence of a watch, the existence of a purposive designer. But why, from his point of view, could the watch not be a natural object, one which grows on trees (let us suppose that all the bits are made from wood), and which, if it serves a purpose at all, serves some quite different purpose (perhaps it is a seed), but which, as a *matter of fact*, reacts to the position of the sun and so measures the passage of time? If someone were presented with a pine cone, and discovered, perhaps accidentally, that it reacts to the amount of water vapour in the air and so measures the humidity, though crudely, would he be entitled to conclude that pine cones were made for the purpose of measuring humidity?

The analogy is even more misleading. For the man who is presented with the watch is already standing outside the system and sees it from a privileged position. But if the analogy were exact, if we were to consider his position in relation to the watch as being similar to our position in relation to the universe, then he would have to be one of the parts. What inferences about order, design and purpose could be justifiably drawn from that vantage point?

Of course, the analogy is not part of the argument but simply an illustrative device which is intended to lend persuasive support to it. That there is something wrong with the analogy, therefore, is not to say that there is something wrong with the argument. What the analogy does reveal, however, is that the argument is deceptively simple. The crucial assertion in it is that order is indicative of a design; but that is not a simple claim, and it is difficult to see how it could be justified except in analogical terms. If the claim rests on evidence, then it rests on our experience of orders which reveal designs within the universe. Yet we have to interpret the claim in such a way that it applies to the universe as a whole; and that seems to be an analogical interpretation.

That there is a universe; that there are causal relationships within it; these two facts by themselves seem to be inadequate as evidence for the existence of God – or even of a god who is either the creator, the designer or both, whatever other properties he might have. Nevertheless, it might be said, there is evidence, much more specific than these two facts, which points to the existence of a god with the power to intervene in wordly events. But it seems not unreasonable to believe, if only on the grounds of economy, that a god with such a power is also both the designer and creator. Such a being is at least close to the idea we have of God, especially so if the interventions are beneficial to us, for the being is then a benevolent god.

Is there any evidence of divine intervention in the causal order? We do speak of miracles and mean by this events which are brought about by a supernatural being; but if we are to turn to miracles as evidence for the existence of a supernatural being, we must have some independent criteria of what it is for an event to be counted as a miracle. It would be idle to argue that because miracles are brought about by a supernatural being, so there must be such a being to bring them about. We first have to show that some events are miracles, independently of the appeal to a supernatural being. We cannot know that there are or are not miracles unless we have criteria for deciding whether or not an event is a miracle.

Suppose we say that a miracle is an event which is not merely unexplained but is in principle inexplicable in natural terms. The fact that we fail to find a satisfactory explanation of an event, does not of course imply that it is inexplicable. To establish such a conclusion, we need to show that there *could not be* a natural explanation, that the event cannot in principle be explained. But how could we ever show this? We might perhaps say that an event is inexplicable in natural terms if it somehow goes against the natural order. But does this mean that it violates a particular natural law or that it violates one or more of the general principles of causation?

Events which violate natural laws are not uncommon; but neither are they inexplicable, at least not usually. Suppose somebody takes a massive dose of arsenic, enough to kill a regiment, but feels no ill-effects. Would that be a miracle? It would be a surprising event, an extraordinary event, an event without precedent. But what, in the end, would justify our saying that it was a miraculous event? Such an event would not put a stop to causal enquiry; on the contrary, it would stimulate it. We should want to know why the man failed to die; and in seeking an answer to this we might well discover a great many new facts about human physiology which explain the man's immunity to arsenic. Of course we might not; but at what point do we give up and say there *cannot be* a natural explanation? There is a general law that arsenic kills human beings when taken in sufficient quantities, but that only holds under appropriate conditions and it is always open to us to say that the conditions are unusual and to seek an explanation why. And even if our enquiry turns up nothing unusual, that would not of itself be grounds for classifying the event as miraculous. It would only be grounds for saying that we do not yet know enough about human physiology to explain what has happened. We can always put the lack of an explanation down to our lack of knowledge.

But some events might be so bizarre that they defeat the possibility of an explanation within the science in which they would normally be explained. If tears come from the eyes of a wooden statue at a particular time of a particular day every year, we might say that there is no possibility of a natural explanation. For an ordinary causal account of crying is in terms of glands, tear ducts, and the rest; but the statue has none of these. But does this mean that there can be *no* causal explanation? Clearly there could not be a causal explanation in physiological terms, but we need only suppose that this is the kind of explanation we should seek if we interpret drops of liquid coming from carved eyes on a piece of wood as tears. They are, however, simply drops of liquid, even though they have the same chemical composition as tears, and they are oozing out of wood. And why is that *in principle* inexplicable? Perhaps the chemist will be able to give us an explanation which the physiologist is in principle unable to give.

We can of course always deny the possibility of a miracle by denying the reported facts. We could say that Christ did not turn the water into wine but simply used mass hypnotism to induce in people the belief that he did; or that he did not rise from the dead because he was not really dead, people simply believed mistakenly that he was. But this is not the point at issue. The question is whether, given that certain extraordinary events did occur, we can find some criteria in terms of which we can justify saying that they are or are not miraculous. It is not the historical question of whether there have or have not been extraordinary events.

Yet however extraordinary the events, it seems that by exercising our ingenuity we can always think up a possible natural explanation. Of course, in seeking to propose natural explanations of extra-ordinary events, it is inevitable that the explanations will often appear to be as bizarre as the events themselves. For unless the enquiry is seriously scientific, it can only be speculative. That by stretching the imagination we can concoct possible explanations, however, is illustrative of the fact that no violation of a natural law could count as a miracle since our procedures of enquiry guarantee a permanent possibility of explanation. When a law fails, we are committed by our procedures to look for the cause of the failure and the mere fact that we do not find one could never be decisive in establishing that there could not be one. These procedures derive from the belief that every spatio-temporal event has at least a temporal cause and the complementary belief that the same cause will, under the same conditions, produce the same effect. A natural law is simply the expression of a cause-effect relationship relatively to certain conditions; so if the law fails, we can simply say that the conditions are not right, and then, using the principle that every event has a cause, look for the cause which affected the conditions. And this technique has no limitations. It may not in particular cases actually lead us to an adequate explanation, but at the same time it blocks the conclusion that there could not be one.

If there are miracles, then, they must be events which violate one or other, or both, of these principles, and not just events which violate natural laws. And it is clear that an event which violated the principle that every spatio-temporal event has at least a temporal cause would, if it has a cause at all, be a miracle. For to say that there are such events is effectively to say that some spatio-temporal events have a non-spatial and non-temporal cause. But that is just what a miracle would be: an event which occurs as the result of a cause outside the spatio-temporal order.

So if there are such events, we can indeed say that there could not be a natural explanation of them; they would be in principle inexplicable. But this does not of course tell us that there *are* such events. Instead we now have the problem of finding some criterion for determining when such an event occurs. And in fact we could never decide whether an event was or was not of this kind without *first* abandoning the principle that every event does have at least a temporal cause. For whenever an event occurs, either we use the principle to justify saying that it has a natural cause, even if we cannot find it, in which case we pre-judge the question of its miraculousness; or we do not use the principle, in which case we beg the question of its miraculousness. There is no way out of this.

But it might be said that we arrive at this dilemma only because we started off on the wrong foot. We were wrong to characterise miracles as events which are in principle inexplicable in natural terms, for God may work his miracles by way of natural causes. In this case, however, how do we distinguish a natural cause-effect relationship which is miraculous from one which is not? Or are we to say that God's actions are a supplementary cause of every event?

It now begins to seem, in general, that if there is evidence for the existence of God, we could never recognise it as such. For our techniques of enquiry do not provide for the possibility of causes outside the spatio-temporal universe, and events which are explicable in terms of causes within it do not require an action from God as a supplementary cause. But if this is so, then arguments for the existence of God which depend on an appeal to worldly evidence cannot succeed.

It may nevertheless be thought that arguments against the existence of God, which also make an appeal to worldly evidence can succeed. For if the facts of the world are such as to be incompatible with any being's having the properties of God, then since the universe is as it is, God does not exist. If, for example, it is held that God is all-powerful, and if we recognise that there is evil in the world, then God is not wholly good; alternatively, if God is wholly good, then the fact of evil in the world shows that he is not all-powerful. Hence God, conceived of as an all-powerful wholly good being, does not exist – though it is of course left open whether a god with only one of these properties, together with all other properties of God, exists.

We might seek to meet this argument by denying the facts; by saying, for example, that there is no evil in the world. But that seems perverse. Or we might seek to meet it by saying that the evil in the world is a consequence of man's actions, not God's. But this, too, seems perverse since the suffering and consequential evil arising from natural disasters, such as earthquakes, are certainly not the result of man's actions. And even that evil which does result from the actions of men could be prevented by an all-powerful god. It may be said, perhaps, that such interventions would prevent men from exercising their freedom of choice and this freedom is in itself wholly good. So if God interfered here, he would be taking away a good in order to prevent an evil. Bu why not? To prevent a particular man from deciding to torture and then massacre a whole community is, in ordinary human terms at least, a far better thing to do than to refrain from interfering simply on the ground that he ought to be left free to make his own decisions. But whatever answer is given here, nothing can change the fact that some suffering is not caused by men; yet any good man who had the power to prevent it would do so, so why not God if he is both omnipotent and benevolent? No doubt there are straws to be clutched at here. We might say that God's ways are mysterious and beyond our comprehension; that his purpose in allowing suffering may be wholly good; that those who suffer in this life will be rewarded in the next; and so on. But if we claim these things in order to reconcile the existence of suffering with the existence of an omnipotent and benevolent god, we are effectively destroying what conception we might seem to have of God's properties. For if omnipotence and benevolence are not to-gether incompatible with the fact of suffering, whatever God's grand design, they are not extensions of our ordinary concepts of power and good and they are, therefore, empty.

Yet though the argument carries some conviction, it is not clear that it has any more strength than arguments in favour of the existence of God. For it depends on the presupposition that there are situations in the universe where God could have intervened but did not. But if it is the case that we cannot know what would count as evidence of a divine intervention, then there never is a situation of which we could say that God has or has not intervened. With what justification, then, can we say that God is not all-powerful because he has not intervened, or that he is not wholly good because he has not intervened? It is not enough simply to say that whenever evil occurs in a particular situation there has been no intervention. For suppose there are cases where God has intervened to prevent evil, then the non-evil events which occurred are inexplicable in ordinary causal terms. Yet we would never recognise them as such. So how could we recognise a situation in which an intervention has taken place – whatever qualities it may have, whether, that is, it is evil or not?

But perhaps we can say *in general*, rather than of particular situations, that there would be no evil at all if a good all-powerful god existed. So it is simply the existence of evil, or more particularly of suffering, which carries the argument; and indeed this is where its force lies even though we can never point to a particular situation and say of it that no intervention took place here. Nevertheless, it is not clear what is meant by saying that there is evil, or that evil in general exists, which could have been prevented by an omnipotent god, if not that there are evil situations in which no divine intervention took place.

What are we to conclude from all of this? The arguments considered here which claim to establish the existence of God on the basis of evidence of what goes on in the universe are at best inconclusive, at worst incomprehensible. Though they may seem to make sense, they do so in fact only if we are prepared to extend the idea of a cause, derived from experience, beyond the possibility of experience. They are not of course the only arguments, nor even the only arguments which purport to rest on evidence. There are, for example, those who claim to have direct acquaintance of God in religious experience, and it might seem that this is a comprehensible claim, though it may be false. For just as we are directly aware of our thoughts, even though we do not perceive them and they are not in space, so it is possible that we could be directly aware of God's thoughts, and so of God. But here, too, there is a presupposition that we have criteria, or that we could establish criteria, which enable us to discriminate those of our mental experiences which are truly ours and those which are caused by God. And it seems in general that any argument which rests on evidence must make a similar presupposition. It must, that is, presuppose that we have or could have clear criteria for recognising the occurrence of certain events, whether mental or physical, *as constituting evidence* for the existence of God. Yet how could there be criteria of this kind if the events are themselves worldly and are nevertheless to stand as evidence which takes us beyond the possibility of experience? But if arguments for the existence of God are not based on evidence, if instead they rest only on conceptions of what we presume God's properties to be, then they are inevitably fallacious since existence cannot be established on the basis of properties alone.

Yet arguments against the existence of God, though we have considered only one, seem to exhibit similar misconceptions. For if they rest on evidence, they presuppose that we have criteria which enable us to classify certain events *as constituting evidence* against the existence of God. To say that an event counts as evidence against, however, is usually to imply that it fails to count as evidence for, and this seems to presuppose that we have a clear understanding of what it is for an event to count as evidence for. But again, if the arguments do not rest on evidence, then, like those in favour of God's existence, they cannot succeed.

Even so, if every argument which claims to establish the existence of God is inevitably fallacious, it does not follow that he does not exist. And if every argument which claims to establish that God does not exist is inevitably fallacious, it does not follow that he does exist. How could we in any case expect to establish the existence or non-existence of a non-spatio-temporal being on any basis whatever? What is beyond the possibility of experience is beyond our comprehension. If God does exist, we cannot know it; and if he does not, we cannot know that either.

FURTHER READING

This is not in any way intended as a complete bibliography. It is simply a list of follow-up suggestions including some recent works as well as historical sources. In choosing recent books and articles, I have tried to select those which do not presuppose much background in philosophy and which either excel in the presentation of a particular problem or take the problem a stage further. These restrictions, especially the first, have excluded many important books. However, those who get to the end of this list will have found plenty of other references to chase up. Entries are listed under each chapter in a recommended order of reading.

Chapter 1

HUME, David: *An Enquiry Concerning Human Understanding*, Section VII, in *Hume's Enquiries*, ed. L. A. Selby-Bigge, Clarendon Press, Oxford, Second edn., 1902.

MILL, John Stuart: *A System of Logic*, Book III, Ch. 5; Book VI, Ch. 2, Longmans, Green & Co., 1843.

COLLINGWOOD, R. G.: 'On the So-called Idea of Causation', *Proceedings of the Aristotelian Society*, 1938.

GASKING, D. A. T.: 'Causation and Recipes', *Mind*, 1957.

Chapter 2

RUSSELL, Bertrand: *The Problems of Philosophy*, Ch. VI, Home University Library, Williams & Northgate, London, 1912. (OPUS edn., 1967.)

EDWARDS, Paul: 'Bertrand Russell's Doubts about Induction' in *Logic and Language*, First Series, ed. A. G. N. Flew, B. H. Blackwell, Oxford, 1951.

WILL, Frederick: 'Will the Future Be Like the Past?' *Mind*, 1948.

Chapter 3

RUSSELL, Bertrand: *The Problems of Philosophy*, Chs. I–IV incl., Home University Library, Williams & Northgate, London, 1912. (OPUS edn., 1967.)

AYER, A. J.:   *The Central Questions of Philosophy*, Ch. IV, Weidenfeld and Nicolson, London, 1973.

DESCARTES, R.:   *Discourse on Method*, Parts II and IV; and *Meditations*, Parts I, II, V and VI; both in *Descartes, A Discourse on Method, etc.*, Everyman, London, 1912.

LOCKE, John: *Essay on the Human Understanding*, Book II, Chs. 1–9 incl. and Ch. 23, ed. A. D. Woozley, Fontana Library, London, 1964.

BERKELEY, G.:   *Three Dialogues between Hylas and Philonous*; and *Principles of Human Knowledge*, Introduction and Part I; both in *Berkeley, New Theory of Vision, etc.*, Everyman, London, 1910.

HUME, David: *Treatise of Human Nature*, Book I, Part IV, Section 2, ed. D. G. C. MacNabb, Fontana Library, London, 1962.

AYER, A. J.:   *The Foundations of Empirical Knowledge*, Macmillan, 1962.

PRICE, H. H.:   *Perception*, Methuen, London, 1932.

MUNDLE, C. W. K.:   *Perception: Facts and Theories*, Oxford University Press, OPUS Series, 1971.

ARMSTRONG, D. M.:   *Perception and the Physical World*, Routledge and Kegan Paul, London, 1961.

Chapter 4

AYER, A. J.:   *The Central Questions of Philosophy*, Ch. VI, Weidenfeld and Nicolson, London, 1973.

DESCARTES, R.:   *Discourse on Method*, Part V; and *Meditations*, Part II; both in *Descartes, A Discourse on Method, etc.*, Everyman, London, 1912.

LOCKE, John: *Essay on the Human Understanding*, Book II, Chapter 21, section 2 and Chapter 23, sections 15, 20 and 28; Book IV, Chapter 9; ed, A. D. Woozley, Fontana Library, London, 1964.

HUME, David: *Treatise of Human Nature*, Book I, Part IV, Section 6, ed. D. G. C. MacNabb, Fontana Library, London, 1962.

RYLE, Gilbert: *The Concept of Mind*, Hutchinson, London, 1949.

SMART, J. J. C.:   'Sensations and Brain-Processes', *Philosophical Review*, 1959.

ARMSTRONG, D. M.:   *A Materialist Theory of the Mind*, Routledge and Kegan Paul, London, 1968.

Chapter 5

HUME, David:
An Enquiry Concerning Human Understanding, Sections VII and VIII, in *Hume's Enquiries*, ed. L. A. Selby-Bigge, Clarendon Press, Oxford, second edn., 1902.

MOORE, G. E.:
Ethics, Ch. 6, Oxford University Press, London, 1912.

CAMPBELL, C. A.:
In Defence of Free-Will, Jackson, Son & Co., Glasgow, 1938.

HART, H. L. A. & HONORE, A. N.:
Causation in the Law, Clarendon Press, Oxford, 1959.

MORRIS, Herbert (ed.):
Freedom and Responsibility, Stanford University Press, California, 1961.

LEHRER, Keith (ed.):
Freedom and Determinism, Harper & Row, New York, 1966.

HART, H. L. A.:
'The Ascription of Responsibility and Rights' in *Logic and Language*, First Series, ed. A. G. N. Flew, B. H. Blackwell, Oxford, 1951.

Chapter 6

DESCARTES, R.:
Discourse on Method, Part IV; and *Meditations*, Part III; both in *Descartes, A Discourse on Method, etc.*, Everyman, London, 1912.

HUME, David:
Dialogues Concerning Natural Religion, ed. with an introduction by N. K. Smith, Nelson, London, second edn., 1947; and *An Enquiry Concerning Human Understanding*, Section X, ed. L. A. Selby-Bigge, Clarendon Press, Oxford, second edn., 1902.

MILL, John Stuart:
Three Essays on Religion, Longmans, Green & Co., 1874; and *An Examination of Sir William Hamilton's Philosophy*, Ch. 7, Longmans, Green & Co., 1865.

WISDOM, John:
'Gods' in *Philosophy and Psycho-Analysis*, Blackwell, Oxford, 1957.

HICK, John:
The Existence of God, Macmillan, 1964.

PIKE, Nelson:
God and Evil: Readings on the Theological Problems of Evil, Prentice Hall, 1964.

TAYLOR, A. E.:
Does God Exist? Macmillan, 1945.